Core Oral Surgery for Dental Students

Second Edition

Essential Knowledge for Qualifying Dentistry Examinations

Andrew Sadler, Judith Jones and Edmund Bailey

All Rights Reserved

First Published   2018.

This edition 2024

Core Oral Surgery for Dental Students

ISBN: 978-1-7393838-3-1

Preface

Core Oral Surgery is designed to help undergraduate dental students in the United Kingdom, and in other countries which follow a similar curriculum, to understand the basic oral surgery knowledge needed for clinical practice in primary care dentistry and most particularly what is required from them in their qualifying examinations. The text adheres to the requirement of the General Dental Council document 'Preparing for Practice' and the newer guidance 'Safe Practitioner Framework'.

The book is also aimed at candidates taking the Overseas Registration Examination of the General Dental Council as that examination requires a performance equivalent to the 'just passed' standard in UK universities. We believe it may act as an aide memoire for established practitioners wanting to review current practice.

Chapters 01 to 05 provide background information which students should be familiar with before they approach patients in the clinical situation; chapters 06 to 13 are concerned with the practical aspects of procedures the student will be expected to undertake; chapters 14 to 16 are concerned with anaesthesia and 17 to 24 conditions that are managed surgically which the student would be expected to have knowledge of but not necessarily treat themselves.

Second Edition

For the second edition the book has been revised and updated to reflect changes in practice and to update new guidances in the surgical management of oral conditions.

July 2024

Acknowledgements

We would like to acknowledge the help and cooperation of the following colleagues in the preparation of this book:

Richard Thornton: - Anaesthesia & sedation

Sarah Bourne: - Radiography

Mital Patel: - Dental trauma

Leo Cheng - Patient examination, odontogenic cysts and tumours

Michael Davidson - Odontogenic cysts and tumours

Tom Sheehan - Radiotherapy and chemotherapy

Contents

01 Taking a History, Examining and Presenting a Patient

Taking a history with particular significance to oral surgery

Taking a sound history in a methodical and consistent manner is the bedrock of diagnosis and therefore of patient management. You should also learn to present patients to tutors and colleagues in an accepted order before management is discussed. You will need to do this in clinical examinations.

You should take the opportunity to carry out both these tasks in the oral surgery clinic whenever you contemplate a dental extraction. Each time you present a patient to a tutor you should consider it to be practice for an examination.

Here is the generally accepted format for history taking.

1. Patient's presenting complaint. (C/O). The symptoms they describe, the signs they report to you or the reason they are seeking treatment.

2. History of presenting complaint. (HPC). The past history of the presenting complaint.

3. Past medical history (PMH). Their current medical status, past serious illnesses, previous surgery.

4. Medication (Med). A list of any medication they are taking or have taken regularly in the past.

5. Allergies. To any medication they have had in the past, any food allergies. Any asthma, hay fever or eczema.

6. Past dental history (PDH). Previous dental treatment and whether they are regular dental attenders and their attitude to conserving their teeth.

7. Social History. Their occupation, alcohol and tobacco consumption and any social factors related to their dental treatment.

Extra oral examination

We wonder how many dentists carry out an extra oral examination of their patients in practice. However you will be expected to do it in your examinations so this is what is expected:

1. Examine the face for obvious asymmetry or swelling. → Asymmetry may be caused by trauma, the soft tissues may be swollen from it, the zygomatic prominence may be flat if the zygoma [cheek] is fractured, and the mandible may be asymmetric if broken. There may be asymmetry in congenital deformities or TMJ growth problems. Mouth opening may be asymmetric due to trauma or internal derangement of the TMJ i.e. disc displacement. The soft tissues may be swollen with oedema from acute inflammation resulting from dental infection; this will be soft swelling or may be firm if there is a collection of pus. There may be swelling from intra oral tumours, particularly squamous cancer or from squamous cancer of the antrum. Benign tumour of the salivary glands will present with swelling.

2. Observe the facial skin for suspicious lesions. → You may be the first to observe a basal cell carcinoma of the skin (locally invasive but not metastasising), a squamous carcinoma or a dark patch which might be malignant melanoma (very malignant). These are more common in those with sun damaged skin who have been outdoors a lot.

3. Palpate the neck and submandibular triangle for swelling, lymphadenopathy and enlargement of submandibular salivary glands. → Firm swelling of the neck lymph nodes may represent metastatic squamous cancer of the mouth or elsewhere in the upper aero-digestive tract. Softer swelling may indicate infection draining. Rubbery enlargement may be due to lymphoma. Small children are susceptible to very

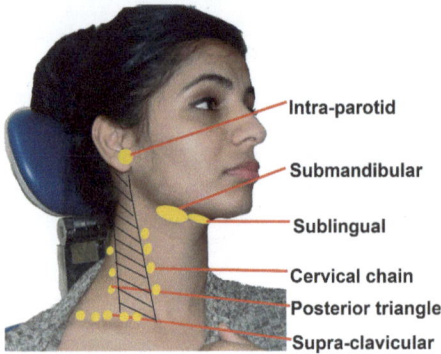

Cervical lymph nodes in relation to sternomastoid muscle

frequent upper respiratory tract infections and they frequently have enlarged cervical nodes with no sinister connotations. If the submandibular gland is enlarged it is best palpated bi-manually with a finger on the superficial surface in the submandibular triangle and a gloved finger on the deep part in the mouth. Swelling may indicate a stone (hard), an infection which is often secondary to a stone obstruction (tender) or a tumour (rare). Salivary tumours may be benign or malignant (chapter 22).

4. Palpate the parotid glands. → The parotid glands may be swollen from infection (tender), tumour (firm) which are most commonly benign, or because the intra-glandular lymph nodes are enlarged (rare) which can be metastatic cancer (from the ear). Ask about previous skin surgery.

5. Palpate the temporomandibular joints (TMJ) while the patient opens their mouth and record any clicking or crepitus. Measure their mouth opening as interincisal distance. → Patients with internal derangement of the TMJ may have their symptoms exacerbated by prolonged mouth opening for dental treatment. They should be warned of this and their pre-treatment condition recorded.

6. Neurology. We don't think it is reasonable to expect dentists to examine the function of the cranial nerves but in the event of fractures or swelling record any numbness of the lip/mental area or

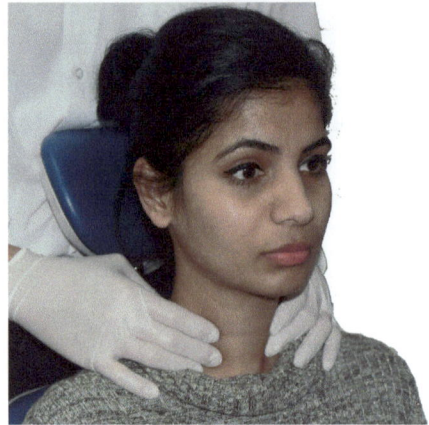

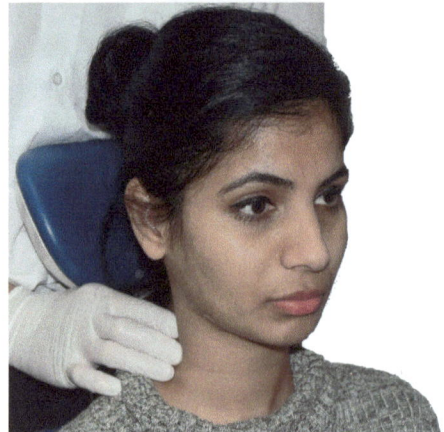

Palpation of the neck for cervical lymphadenopathy

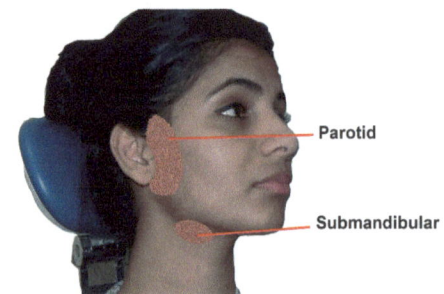

Position of the submandibular and parotid salivary glands

infraorbital region. → Decreased sensation of the lip/mental area is most common after previous surgery but can occur as a result of fracture of the mandible (although it usually recovers) and rarely may be a presenting feature of intra bony malignancy or cyst (chapter 20). Decreased sensation of the infra

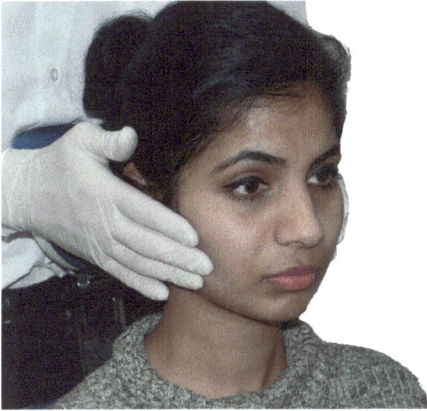

Palpate the parotid glands for generalised enlargement or discreet lumps

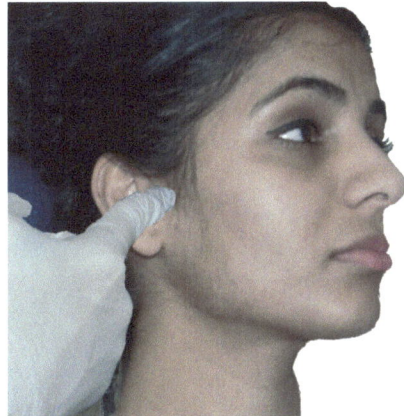

Palpate the temporo mandibular joints during opening and closing and note clicking, crepitation or asymmetric movement

orbital nerve is most commonly due to nerve compression in a fracture of the zygoma, although it usually recovers, but can be due to carcinoma of the antrum. Look for swelling of the face and palpate for expansion of the buccal sulcus. Any paraesthesia or anaesthesia of these sensory nerves should be considered as a sinister sign of malignancy unless there is a simpler explanation of some form of trauma to the nerve.

Intra oral examination

1. Observe the lips for obvious swelling. → Thickening of vermillion of lower lip, actinic chelitis (sun damage which is potentially pre-cancerous) ulceration from squamous cancer, soft swelling within the lip - mucous cyst.

2. Retract the lips and examine the buccal mucosa each side and if any abnormality is seen palpate with a gloved finger. → White or red patches anywhere in oral mucosa may indicate a potentially malignant condition.

3. Examine the floor of the mouth and if any abnormality seen palpate. → Sublingual keratosis is a potentially malignant disorder. Swelling of sublingual gland is rare but tumours are more likely to be malignant than in other salivary glands.

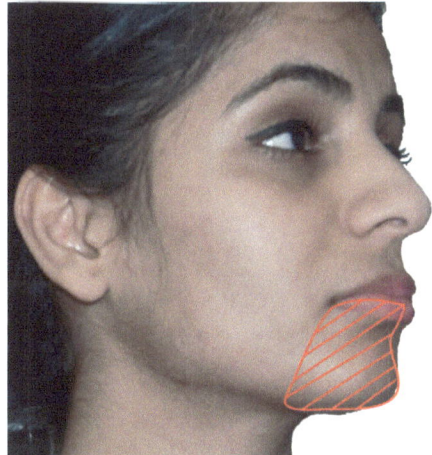

The mental distribution where sensation may be compromised in injury to the inferior dental nerve by fracture, surgery or rarely malignant tumour

4. Examine and palpate the sulci and alveolus upper and lower, buccal and lingually. → Swelling related to minor salivary glands or swelling of alveolus may represent a cyst, intra bony tumour or dental abscess. A sinus may be draining from a chronically infected tooth.

5. Examine the tongue. Pull it forward, holding it with a surgical swab at the tip, and palpate it on both lateral margins. → Look for white patches or small squamous cell carcinoma on lateral margin of tongue. Be aware of appearance of lingual

3

tonsillar tissue, which patients are often worried about if they notice it, and circumvallate papillae at junction of anterior and posterior third of tongue. Tumours on the dorsum of the tongue are very rare.

6. Depress the tongue with a mouth mirror and examine the tonsillar/oropharyngeal area.

7. Examine the teeth for caries and periodontal disease.

8. Note any over-erupted teeth or abnormalities of occlusion.

Presenting a patient

You should get plenty of practice of presenting cases to your tutors in the clinic before extracting teeth. You will need to do this in examinations and future professional team working. Before any extraction you should take a history yourself, examine the patient, draw up a treatment plan (even when these steps have already been done by others). Consider any alternative management and particularly why the tooth is not to be restored and present the case to a tutor.

Patients should be presented in a logical order which is the universally accepted and practised way within the dental and medical professions. This gets the points over briefly and methodically so that a colleague can easily join in a discussion about the patient's management.

1. Introduce the patient with their name, age, occupation and what treatment is proposed or the problem they presented with.

Then proceed in the same order as history taking.

2. What their symptoms are.

3. History of their presenting symptoms (briefly).

4. Medical history or absence of any. Report specific negative findings only if

relevant. (e.g. report that they are not taking any medication which might promote bleeding only if bleeding is their problem).

5. Medication.

6. Allergies.

7. Social history, tobacco use or its absence is relevant to almost all oral care.

8. Examination findings, again report negative findings only if relevant.

9. Special investigations. Report all that have been done and their negative findings (if they were irrelevant we assume they wouldn't have been carried out).

10. Diagnosis or differential diagnosis if the diagnosis is uncertain.

11. Proposed treatment.

12. One sentence summary.

Example:

"This is Mr George Hansel who is a 64 retired plumber who has been referred from the urgent dental clinic for removal of lower right 6. Mr Hansel has severe pain from the right mandible which started as a dull ache a week ago following a few weeks of sensitivity to hot and cold and yesterday he reported swelling over the mandible.

Mr Hansel has type 2 diabetes which is well controlled by diet. He takes no medication and has no known allergies. He has not received regular dental treatment. He attends only when he has problems.

On examination he is partly dentate with no prostheses, the lower right first molar is carious, tender to percussion and slightly mobile. There is oedematous swelling over the mandible.

A periapical radiograph shows caries and apical radiolucency. Diagnosis is acute alveolar abscess lower right 6, he does not want restoration. The plan is to remove the tooth now with local anaesthetic."

Cranial Nerves (for reference)

1: Olfactory - smell

2: Optic - sight

3: Oculomotor - eye movement

4: Trochlear - eye movement

5: Trigeminal - sensation head, neck and face; motor masticatory muscles

6: Abducens - eye movement

7: Facial - motor muscles of facial expression; sensation anterior tongue and tympanic membrane

8: Vestibulocochlear - hearing and balance

9: Glossopharyngeal - motor swallowing; sensory posterior tongue, pharynx

10: Vagus - sensation, motor and autonomic to viscera

11: Spinal accessory - head movement

12: Hypoglossal - movement of tongue

Examination tips:

- Use every opportunity to take histories and present patients so that it is automatic and second nature to you by the time you get to your examinations.

- If you are asked to take a history in an OSCE (objective structured clinical examination) you will be given marks for taking the history and asking relevant questions in a methodical manner not just for finding out the problems and making a diagnosis.

- You usually get marks by introducing yourself and being nice to the 'patient' (who will be an actor in an OSCE).

- You usually get marks for good hygiene i.e. being bare below the elbows and washing your hands before the examination.

- Always record the diagnosis.

02 Patient Assessment - Potential Medical Problems

In this chapter we will consider the medical problems which may affect decisions made in treatment planning oral surgery. These are listed in the table. Of course there are a large number of medical issues which may theoretically impinge on dentistry but we have limited ourselves to the ones that may make a difference in everyday clinical practice and/or that you may be expected to know about for your examinations. We have included general medical problems and local mouth related issues but not medical emergencies or resuscitation (see guidelines Appendix 3).

Recent cardiac events

Following a myocardial infarction, non ST elevation myocardial infarction, acute coronary syndrome or unstable angina a patient may have an irritable myocardium and will be at increased risk of another adverse cardiac event or infarction. It is usually recommended that extraction should be postponed for a period of six months after such an event unless it cannot be avoided due to, for example, an acute abscess. There may be a risk of reinfarction which will be higher if there are comorbidities such as older age, obesity, diabetes, or a history of stroke and lower if the patient is taking statins or anticoagulants or has been treated with a coronary artery stent. Treatment may be delayed for only 4 to 6 weeks if a stent has been fitted.

These patients may well be taking anticoagulants and antiplatelet medication. Some will have been fitted with a drug-eluting stent in a coronary artery in which case they may be taking an anticoagulant together with aspirin or clopidogrel which both decrease platelet 'stickiness' in order to decrease the risk of thrombosis. They will have an increased risk of bleeding following extraction but a very real risk of thrombosis of the stent if any of the medication is stopped so urgent extractions to control acute infection must

---

> ### *Medical issues to consider before minor oral surgery*
>
> - cardiac events and hypertension
> - recent stroke
> - diabetes
> - steroids
> - coagulation disorders
> - anticoagulants
> - antiplatelet medication
> - other medication compromising clotting
> - liver disease
> - medication associated with jaw necrosis
> - local radiotherapy
> - temporomandibular joint
> - Inherited blood disorders
> - Respiratory disease

---

proceed without ceasing the medication and their cardiologist should be consulted.

Local measures should be used to decrease the risk of bleeding which include suturing the socket and packing with oxidised cellulose gauze. Non-steroidal anti-inflammatory medications should not be used for analgesia as they may encourage bleeding (Chapter 12). The drug of choice for pain relief should usually be paracetamol.

Recent Stroke

Any form of surgery including dental extraction will lead to a slight increasing in blood coagulability. Most strokes are the result of emboli of thrombus within the cerebral circulation and thus surgery can promote further clots. Routine dental extraction should therefore be delayed and advice taken after any thrombotic stroke. Patients may be taking anticoagulants as may patients who have Transient Ischemic Attacks (mini strokes) who are at risk of thrombosis consequent on atrial fibrillation.

Diabetes

A poorly controlled diabetic may exhibit delayed wound healing and have an increased risk of cardio-vascular complications; post-operative infection is more likely. For minor oral surgery you are unlikely to notice any difference in practice. It is also unlikely that dental extraction will influence their calorie intake sufficiently to upset their diabetic regime, particularly if not using general anaesthesia.

If a patient attends for extraction and has been unable to eat and has taken their normal insulin there is a possibility of hypoglycemia. Symptoms can develop quickly which are usually sweating, shakiness, tachycardia and anxiety; most patients will recognize the symptoms themselves. Hypoglycemia can be quickly be reversed with a glucose or high sugar drink.

Patients with severe infection may have a 'stress' response sufficient to potentiate catabolic hyperglycemia and ketoacidosis but this will take days to occur and is very unlikely to be a problem in dental practice.

You should bear in mind that the patient who comes with a large dental abscess may be one of the many previously undiagnosed diabetics who are immunocompromised by their condition. Patients with large abscesses should therefore have their glucose levels checked. This can be a simple procedure using a 'finger prick' blood sample in a glucometer.

Steroids

Patients taking long term steroids could theoretically be at risk of their medication causing suppression of their adrenal cortex. This may lead to an inadequate steroid response to metabolic stress leading to Addisonian crisis with hypotension and collapse.

It has often been suggested that these patients have their steroids supplemented at times of stress as prophylaxis against this untoward event. However the risk is low if the patient has been taking 5 mg of prednisolone a day or less has had no steroid for three months.

It is suggested that patients having minor oral surgery and who have had 30 mg or more of prednisolone per day within the last three months should double their morning dose on the day of surgery. Those having major surgery should do the same and have an additional IV dose of hydrocortisone before the procedure. They will probably be having a general anaesthetic so the anaesthetist will give the supplementary hydrocortisone IV and monitor their blood pressure. For some patients under the care of an endocrinologist it is advisable to take their advice.

Patients on long term steroids will have compromised healing and a lowered resistance to infection but this is unlikely to be significant in minor oral surgery. However it is prudent to mention this in examination answers.

Chemotherapy

Chemotherapy is the name given to the use of a variety of anti-cancer drugs for the treatment of malignant conditions, particularly leukaemia and lymphomas, but also some solid tumours such as breast and bowel cancer. Chemotherapy can cause a variety of oral problems which resolve with time. However of specific interest if dental extractions are required is that they cause myelosuppression leading to neutropenia (low white cells), hence a susceptibility to infection. Platelets will also be suppressed and this will frustrate clotting and can lead to prolonged bleeding. In these cases extractions should be delayed for six weeks after chemotherapy treatment when the myelosuppression should have recovered. In the emergency situation the patient should be referred to an oral and maxillofacial surgery department where intravenous antibiotics and/or platelet infusions may be used if extractions cannot be avoided.

Disorders of Haemostasis

You should be aware of the potential problems where haemostasis is compromised, how patients present and what cases to refer to a specialist and who to get help from.

Patients with the commonest disorders: Willebrand disease (due to a hereditary deficiency of von Willebrand factor) which leads to platelet dysfunction, or the Haemophilia (Haemophilia A due to Factor VIII or Haemophilia B factor IX deficiency) will be under the care of a Haemophilia Care Centre. They will know the patient's details and their latest blood results and must be informed about any intended dental extractions.

Usually extractions for patients with disorders of haemostasis are performed in an oral and maxillofacial or oral surgery department in the hospital where their haematologist is based. However in many cases this is not essential but extractions should only be carried out with the knowledge of their haematologist. They will probably prescribe DDAVP (1-deamino- 8-d-arginine vasopressin) which increases the activity of Factor VIII and promotes release of Von Willebrand Factor and also tranexamic acid, an antifibrinolytic, which frustrates clot breakdown. These are usually taken orally for a few days, starting pre-op. If their clotting factors are particularly low they may be supplemented intravenously.

Patients with a history of idiopathic thrombocytopenia, liver disease (which may affect synthesis of clotting factors) or severe autoimmune disease (which can lead to circulating anticoagulants) should have a medical referral and a blood count to check platelet levels and a coagulation screen before extractions.

In an examination you should repeat the often repeated cliché that the extraction

should be carried out as atraumatically as possible; but when have we ever tried to do the opposite? The sockets should be packed with oxidised cellulose gauze and sutured. Topical tranexamic acid may help if it has not been prescribed systemically. Tranexamic acid is not available in the Dental Practitioners Formulary.

Haemophilia is inherited through an X linked recessive gene leading to a deficiency of clotting factor XIII (Haemophilia A) or factor IX (Haemophilia B, Christmas disease); it is thus more common in males. However you should be aware that about 30% of cases may arise from spontaneous mutations so that there may be no family history. New cases may present in childhood with inappropriate bleeding or bruising or, if mild, at the first experience of surgery which may be dental extraction. Rarely haemophilia can be acquired due to the development of autoantibodies. These may present with prolonged bleeding after extraction but give a history of having previous surgery with no problems. The message is that anyone with inappropriate bleeding should be referred for coagulation screening; the patient's GP can arrange this.

Antiplatelet Medication

Aspirin, clopidogrel and dipyridamole are used to prevent platelet adhesion and prevent unwanted vascular events such as acute coronary thrombosis, stroke and transient ischemic attacks. For minor oral surgery such as surgical dental extraction the risk of bleeding which cannot be controlled by local measures is very low; so surgery should proceed without stopping the medication. In some cases where, used in conjunction with cardiac stents, it is dangerous to do so. Extractions can be accompanied by socket packing, suturing and tranexamic acid.

Anticoagulants - Warfarin

Many patients are anticoagulated to reduce the risk of thromboembolism caused by atrial fibrillation, mechanical heart valves or because they are considered high risk because they have had a previous thrombosis.

Warfarin blocks the formation of prothrombin and vitamin K dependant clotting factors. It has a long half-life of about 36 hours which means the full anticoagulant effects take some time to be reached and continue for several days after the medication is stopped.

The degree of anticoagulation is measured with the prothrombin test and is expressed as the INR (International Normalized Ratio) which is the ratio of the prothrombin time divided by a laboratory control. An INR of 1 would be normal, i.e. no anticoagulation, and 2 would mean the blood would take twice as long to clot. Patients have their warfarin doses adjusted to achieve the INR appropriate to the problem they have which might lead to thromboembolism. This will be between 2 and 3 for patients at risk due to atrial fibrillation, a previous deep vein thrombosis, pulmonary embolism or transient ischemic events or strokes. A higher ratio of between 3 and 4 is appropriate for those who are at risk because of heart valve disorders including mechanical heart valves or a recent myocardial infarct.

Patients who are anticoagulated within these therapeutic ranges of INR 2-4 are likely to have some additional risk of bleeding following minor oral surgery including dental extractions. However this is nearly always susceptible to being stopped by simple local measures such as packing, suturing and locally applied tranexamic acid. Stopping the anticoagulation places them at increased risk of rebound thrombosis so it is generally recommended that no adjustment is appropriate if the patient's INR is within the therapeutic range (INR <4).

Patients who take warfarin will have an anticoagulant alert card with all their blood results recorded on it. If they have a stable result dental extractions can be carried out but with the above local measures, but if they have unstable results they should be seen on an anticoagulant clinic and have their dosage adjusted. It is recommended that patients should have their INR checked within 72 hours of extractions.

Warfarin may be potentiated by other medication such as anti-hypertensives, antifungals, carbamazepine, steroids, phenytoin, aspirin, and antibiotics such as erythromycin and metronidazole. In these situations treatment in hospital will give the patient greater confidence that should excess bleeding occur measures will be quickly available to help.

Dentists may prescribe paracetamol, broad spectrum antibiotics (particularly metronidazole) and the antifungals miconazole and fluconazole. These may potentiate warfarin. Sometimes we use steroids after surgery. When prescribing it is wise to always consult the British National Formulary to check for adverse reactions and drug interactions. https://bnf.nice.org.uk/.

Direct Oral Anticoagulants (DOAC) also known as Novel Anticoagulants

Recently newer direct oral anticoagulant drugs, sometimes termed 'target specific' or 'novel' anticoagulants, dabigatran (Pradaxa), rivaroxaban (Xarelto), apixaban (Eliquis) and edoxaban (Lixiana) have become available. They are not antagonists of vitamin K and have certain advantages over warfarin for long term anticoagulation.

The novel anticoagulants have much shorter half-lives than warfarin so they have a more rapid onset of action after oral ingestion and, provided the patient does not have renal failure, a much quicker offset. They have a lower risk of unwanted bleeding, few drug interactions, a much reduced variability of effect between individuals and do not require anticoagulant monitoring; indeed there is no reliable test to do so. There is no effective way of reversing their effect other than by stopping the medication. However idarucizumab, a newer drug, has been recently developed which binds to dabigatran and neutralises its anticoagulant effect and can therefore be used in an emergency situation.

It was only in 2012 that dabigatran received approval from the National Institute of Clinical Excellence for thrombo-prophylaxis for stroke and patients with atrial fibrillation (not accompanied by valve disease). It is therefore too soon for a definitive experience to have been established on how patients taking these drugs should be managed during surgery. However it would appear that patients requiring dental extraction and minor oral surgery do not suffer any major problems if these drugs are continued as normal and provided three or fewer teeth are removed. It is recommended that ideally the surgery should be carried out 12 hours after the last dose; wounds should be sutured.

Other drugs potentiating bleeding

Aspirin will increase bleeding by reducing platelet function but there is no evidence that this will be detrimental in terms of blood loss in oral surgery; any bleeding can be controlled with local measures. The effect is long lasting as aspirin affects platelets for their life and this only decreases as new platelets are formed so that the half-life is several days. Aspirin containing analgesics should therefore not be used by patients having minor oral surgery who are also taking anticoagulants.

Non-steroidal anti-inflammatory drugs such as ibuprofen also decrease platelet function although the effect on the platelets is not permanent and they will recover as the dose wears off. Non-steroidals should also not be used for analgesia in patients taking anticoagulants.

Liver disease

Patients who have severe disease may have clotting problems if they are unable to synthesize clotting factors; also if their disease is related to viral hepatitis there may be an infection risk. If the disease is severe, they may be unable to metabolize and excrete medication satisfactorily. Enquiry should be made about their current status from their general practitioner or physician and an up to date coagulation screen requested if they are to have extractions.

Coagulation Studies

Patients who have had prolonged or excessive bleeding after oral surgery or dental extraction should be investigated with a full blood count to check their platelet count and a coagulation screen.

The coagulation screen consists of three tests: the prothrombin time (PT), activated partial thromboplastin time (APTT) and the thrombin time (TT). If all of these are normal then the coagulation cascade should be normal and produce normal fibrin for haemostasis. If any are abnormal the report

Coagulation Tests

Test	For
Prothrombin time (PT)	Extrinsic coagulation system & final common pathways as it forms fibrin. PT will be normal in Haemophilia A & B as factors VIII & IX are not in the extrinsic system
Activated partial thromboplastin time (APTT)	Intrinsic coagulation system & final common pathway. APTT will be prolonged in Haemophilia A & B as factors VIII & IX are in the intrinsic system
Thrombin time (TT)	Final pathways only. TT will be normal in Haemophilia A & B
International Normalised Ratio (INR)	A ratio of the prothrombin time to a control used to measure the effect of warfarin anticoagulated patients

will advise what to do next: to retest, do additional investigations or to refer the patient to a haematologist. If the patient is still bleeding a haematologist's help will be needed immediately.

Most commonly, clotting factors are deficient due to liver disease, which is acquired. PT will be most sensitive to this but in severe liver disease PT and APTT will both be prolonged; it is unusual for the TT to be affected.

Medication-related Osteonecrosis of the Jaws (MRONJ)

Osteonecrosis of the jaws resulting from bisphosphate medication was first seen in the UK in approximately 2002. It is the same disease that was seen in workers exposed to phosphorus in the match industry in the 19th century. More recently other antiresorptive and antiangiogenic drugs have been found to cause the same disease.

Bisphosphonate medication is prescribed in low doses in oral form to post-menopausal women with osteopenia and osteoporosis to prevent pathological fractures. It can be administered in low dose by six monthly IV infusion for these conditions. It is used in higher dose through intermittent intravenous infusions for the management of Paget's disease of bone, hypercalcaemia of malignancy, multiple myeloma and for skeletal metastases, mostly in women with breast cancer but also men with prostate cancer. Many post-menopausal women will be prescribed bisphosphonates when they are given steroids for any reason. Steroids decrease bone density which increases the risk of osteopenia and osteoporosis in post menopausal women.

The drugs work mainly by inhibiting osteoclastic bone resorption; they are called 'anti-resorptive'. They accumulate in bone, particularly where there is a high bone turn over, as in the alveolus of the jaws. They may also inhibit tumour cells invading bone and cause tumour cell death. It is possible that bisphosphonate may be released from bone by the trauma of dental extractions and thus inhibit soft tissue healing; they may also decrease intra-bony blood circulation. There is a very high turnover of bone during remodelling after dental extraction so that symptoms are most likely to develop in this circumstance.

Osteonecrosis of the jaws has been defined as avascular necrotic bone, which may or may not be exposed, that has been present for over eight weeks in patients with no history of radiation therapy to the jaws or obvious metastatic disease. However, recently a newer drug, denosumab, not a bisphosphonate (a Receptor Activator Nuclear Factor KB Ligand Inhibitor - RANKL), has been introduced. It too is anti-resorptive. This interferes with osteoclast function and has been used for post-menopausal osteoporosis and in some cases replacing bisphosphonate for cancer patients.

Bevacizumab, sunitinib and aflibercept are 'anti-angiogenic' drugs that stop new blood vessel formation and are used in cancer treatment to inhibit tumour growth; they are not anti-resorptive but they may also contribute to necrosis. This has led to the term Medication Related Osteonecrosis of the Jaws (MRONJ) to be used.

Those taking lower dose bisphosphonates mostly orally (commonly alendronic acid) or by six monthly IV infusion are less at risk than those having higher dose intermittent infusions (commonly zoledronic acid). However there are more patients with problems related to low dose use for osteoporosis or osteopenia than high dose due to the much larger number prescribed the former.

Bone necrosis itself can be asymptomatic but when it becomes infected swelling, pain and discharge develop. In most cases this is precipitated by dental extraction although it can rarely occur spontaneously and from denture trauma, particularly on the thin mucosa lingually in the lower molar area or over tori. The longer a patient has been on the medication the greater the risk; most of those on oral bisphosphonate have taken it for five years before getting symptoms.

In most patients who develop bone necrosis which is exposed into the mouth there will be chronic infection with discharge producing a foul smell; they will get intermittent acute exacerbations with swelling and pain. Although this is miserable it is important to remember that these are lifesaving drugs and that, in particular, many women with metastatic breast cancer are able to live relatively normal lives for a prolonged period whereas they might otherwise have been crippled by pathological fractures. Many elderly women have been prevented from having fractures of the neck of femur which itself can be life threatening.

Patients should be made dentally fit before starting the drugs. Any non-restorable teeth should be removed and the socket allowed to heal for three weeks before the first dose. Patients on oral bisphosphonates are at lower risk especially if taking the drug for a short time. They may have extractions carried out as atraumatically as possible and sharp socket edges burred back without raising a muco-periosteal flap. Patients taking oral drugs for over five years and particularly those taking steroids should be warned of higher risk.

Patients on IV bisphosphonates or are at higher risk due to taking medication for five years or more and taking steroids should avoid extractions wherever feasible. For unrestorable teeth removing the crown and root filling the root has been advocated.

The Scottish Dental Clinical Effectiveness Program provides guidance on management (www.sdcep.org.uk).

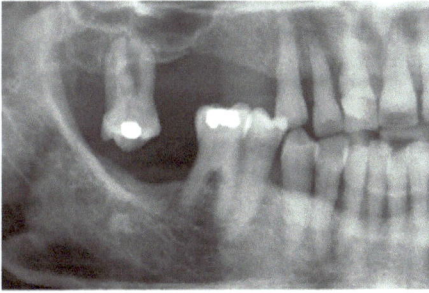

1. *Patient presented with non-functional over-erupted molars which were extracted.*

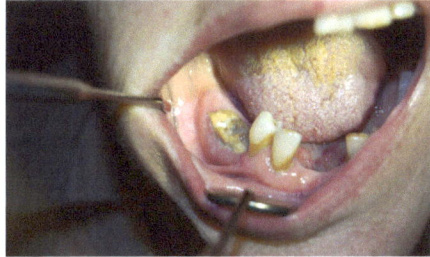

2. *Patient returns with discomfort and foul smell. She was having bisphosphonates.*

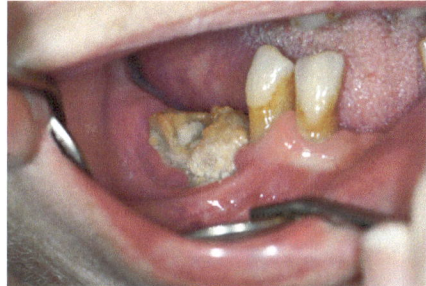

3. *Three months later more bone is visible.*

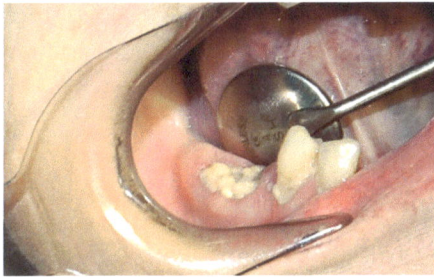

4. *Another six months and it is worse. Eventually the bone may fall out but she will continue to discharge pus for life. Attempts to curette exposed bone will make it worse. Rather than extractions she should have had the crowns removed and the roots filled.*

Drugs causing jaw necrosis
Anti-resorptive: IV Bisphosphonates
zoledronic acid
sodium clodronate
Anti-resorptive: Oral Bisphosphonate
alendronic acid
risedronate sodium
ibandronic acid
Anti-resorptive: RANKL Inbibitor
denosumab
Anti-angiogenic
bevacizumab
sunitinib
aflibercept

Osteoradionecrosis

Radiotherapy uses high energy ionizing radiation to generate free radicals which break double-stranded DNA thus damaging the reproductive activity of cells leading to their death when they attempt to divide at mitosis; they are then removed by the body's own defence mechanism. Normal cells are damaged in the same way as malignant cells but unlike the cancer cells they have the ability to repair; they are thus much less affected.

However the blood supply of the normal tissues is adversely affected by radiotherapy and thus reduces their ability to heal. Intensity Modulated Radiotherapy (IMRT) involves many hundreds of small beams of radiation delivered to the tumour precisely with improved sparing of the normal tissues. It is particularly used for head and neck cancer treatment where there are many structures which will benefit from avoiding radiation, such as the salivary glands, spinal cord and larynx. IMRT has been proved to reduce less long term side effects, particularly the salivary glands reducing xerostomia; radical IMRT is the standard of care that should be provided for head and neck cancer patients.

The most immediate side effect of radiotherapy to the head and neck is mucositis which usually manifests by the second or third week of treatment. It consists of widespread erythema, ulceration bleeding and pain. The oral and pharyngeal mucosa will become inflamed, sore and possibly ulcerated. Maintenance of oral hygiene will be difficult when the mouth is so sore and this may be helped by chlorhexidine mouthwash to help with plaque control. The discomfort will significantly affect the ability to chew and swallow and hence impede nutrition.

The cells of the mucosa exhibit a high rate of turnover so the mucositis can be expected to recover about three weeks after completion of treatment. However radiotherapy will have a permanent effect on the salivary glands, both major and minor, causing permanent damage and dryness of the mouth with such saliva as there is being thick. Whereas the effect is likely to be less with Intensity Modulated Radiotherapy the xerostomia caused will be permanent.

Probably the most serious complication of head and neck radiotherapy results from the effect of radiation on bone, particularly the mandible. The effect of the radiation is to obliterate blood vessels supplying the bone so that it is deprived of nutriments and oxygen. This severely curtails its capacity to remodel, resist infection and heal after trauma.

As with medication induced osteonecrosis the resultant bone necrosis may not be a problem to the patient until the bone is infected, particularly from periodontal or apical dental infection, or is traumatised, particularly by dental extraction. Once infected the necrotic bone will drain pus, become permanently exposed to the mouth and never heal. There will be permanent discharge with discomfort and unpleasant smell. There are likely to be acute exacerbations of the chronic infection with swelling and pain and a risk of pathological fracture.

Recently Pentoxifylline and Tocopherol (vitamin E) have been used in the management of osteonecrosis. It is suggested that together they increase microcirculation in the bone, inhibit inflammation, promote fibroblasts and protect cell membranes. More assessment of this management is needed.

The damage to bone from radiotherapy is permanent so patients are at risk of septic osteoradionecrosis from dental infection or extraction for the remainder of their lives.

It is essential that all patients with oral, nasal or pharyngeal tumours should have a comprehensive assessment of their dentition as soon as they are diagnosed so that they are rendered dentally fit before treatment starts. In most centres the patients are assessed by a restorative dentist which will give the patient the opportunity to discuss future prosthetic rehabilitation. Any dental treatment or assessment should not be allowed to delay cancer treatment. We tend to take a pessimistic approach to future dental health and plan treatment accordingly. In assessing the dentition we acknowledge that most of the patients will be elderly and may have less than ideal periodontal conditions, that they may have less than ideal dental health beforehand.

Radiotherapy will cause xerostomia leading to greatly increased caries risk and that radiotherapy and surgery may lead to some degree of trismus making oral hygiene measures and dental inspection or treatment difficult. This and the experience that osteoradionecrosis is so miserable for the patient usually means we recommend a radical approach and that any teeth which are not completely healthy in terms of tooth substance and periodontium which are in the field of high dose radiation are removed before treatment.

Temporomandibular Joint

Prolonged mouth opening, such as when carrying out a difficult or prolonged dental extraction can exacerbate internal derangement of the temporomandibular joint. Before carrying out any oral surgery it is therefore wise to make a note of any previous symptoms of pain, locking or clicking related to the joint or limitation of mouth opening. The use of a mouth prop during surgery may help reduce the strain on the joint; if the patient finds this uncomfortable it can always be removed.

Inherited blood disorders

Sickle cell disease is caused by an inherited gene (sickle cell trait) which causes an abnormality of haemoglobin and an abnormal shape of the red blood cells. The abnormal cells can cause blockages in the peripheral circulation, anaemia and compromised oxygen carriage.

Thalassemia is a group of disorders of haemoglobin also causing anaemia and compromised oxygen carriage.

These disorders should not necessarily compromise minor oral surgery carried out under local anaesthetic but will be important if a general anaesthetic is contemplated and sedation would would be best administered by a competent anaesthetist.

Respiratory Disease

Chronic obstructive airways disease, COAD, should not adversely affect minor surgery with local anaesthetic although it would be sensible to delay surgery until after any acute exacerbation has settled, as with an acute upper respiratory infection such as the common cold. Patients who are breathless at rest are probably best having extractions carried out with supplementary oxygen through a nasal cannulae supervised by an anaesthetist.

A history of asthma should be noted as it may be exacerbated by stress and must be considered if a general anaesthetic is contemplated. Non steroidal anti-inflammatory medication, which you may prescribe for pain relief, can set off or exacerbate an asthma attack.

Examination tips:

▪ Use your time studying for examinations wisely. For your earlier examinations in human disease and pathology you will be expected to have a greater understanding of medicine but for clinical examinations concentrate more on the essentials covered in this chapter.

▪ In examination answers cover all aspects of the issues presented to you. For example for a question of post extraction bleeding mention the ethical issues of ensuring patients have access to help outside of normal clinic hours.

▪ Always mention to whom and where you would ask for advice or refer a patient with problems you cannot deal with yourself. This shows you are likely to be safe. For example you are unlikely to lose marks for not knowing what coagulation tests should be performed for a patient with persistent bleeding but you will get credit for saying they should be referred for investigation.

▪ Know what equipment and materials are needed in the dental surgery to manage medical problems and emergencies.

03 Consent for Treatment

Before any form of treatment the patient must give their consent. They must be informed what the options are for the clinical problem that they have, what are the benefits, side effects and risk of complications or failure, the likely consequence of no treatment at all and the cost.

The patient must understand what is being offered and be capable of absorbing the information and making choices offered to them. You must take reasonable care to ensure the patient is aware of any material risks involved in treatment and reasonable alternatives and that they have sufficient information to make an informed choice. The patient has a legal

and ethical right to autonomy in making their decision. This is known as the Montgomery principal following a widely reported court case in 2015.

A young person under the age of 16 should be informed about treatment but normally have consent given by a parent. However in rare cases they may wish to receive treatment without their parents' knowledge or consent. In such cases an assessment should be made of their age, maturity, mental capacity, understanding of the treatment and impact, risks, the alternatives and reasoning. If this is all positive, they may be said to be 'Gillick competent' – named after a 1980s court case – and treatment can proceed but they should be encouraged to involve a parent.

The consent form is a useful adjunct to this process but is merely a written confirmation that the process has taken place and is not the end in itself. It should be written in terms that can be understood, so abbreviations and dental notations should not be used. Good clinical notes are important in recording what discussion had taken place and what written information has been given. They are probably of as much use as the consent form itself.

In a very few cases an adult may not be able to understand the issues and does not have the capacity to give consent. In these circumstances they should be treated as defined in the Mental Capacity Act. Here you should get help and advice. It normally involves two clinicians agreeing what treatment is in the patient's best interest in

Barts Health **NHS**
NHS Trust

Consent Form 1

Patient Agreement to Investigation or Treatment

Patient details (or pre-printed label)

Patient's Surname/ Family name...... ++++++ +
Patient's First name...... +++++
Date of Birth.... XX | XX | XXXX
NHS number (or other identifier)......
Sex ☑Male ☐ Female

Responsible health professional ...... Sadler.
Job title ...... Consultant
Special requirements of patient (e.g. language/communication)

Name of proposed procedure or course of treatment (include brief explanation if medical term not clear)
Surgical removal of lower first molar tooth. lower right side.

Statement of health professional (To be filled in by health professional with appropriate knowledge of proposed procedure, as specified in consent policy. It is expected that for all planned procedures consent is obtained prior to the day of treatment).

I have explained the procedure to the patient. In particular, I have explained:
The intended benefits _
Remove pain, prevent abscess

Serious or frequently occurring risks Post extraction pain, swelling, bruising, infection, bleeding. Will need sutures.

Any extra procedures which may become necessary during the procedure
☐ blood transfusion......
☐ other procedure (please specify)......

I have also discussed what the procedure is likely to involve, the benefits and risks of any available alternative treatments (including no treatment) and any particular concerns of this patient.

☐ The following leaflet/tape has been provided......

This procedure will involve:
☐ general and/or regional anaesthesia   ☑local anaesthesia   ☐ sedation
Signed...... A Sadler   Date 26/7/2017
Name (PRINT)...... SADLER   Job title ... Consultant.

Who to Contact (if further information is required or to discuss options later)......

Statement of interpreter (where appropriate)
I have interpreted the information above to the patient to the best of my ability and in a way in which I believe s/he can understand.
Signed......   Date......
Name (PRINT)......

YELLOW COPY: HEALTH RECORDS   BLUE COPY: PATIENT   WHITE COPY: PATHOLOGY

A typical consent form for dental extraction. Remember this only confirms that the consent process has been carried out. Record observations and record any discussion or special issues in the notes. Don't use abbreviations. The patient should sign on the other side.

the light of their examination and information given to them. In English law no adult is able to give consent for another adult, which is rarely understood by well-meaning relatives but they should always be consulted and informed.

You should read and digest the General Dental Council's document - Standards, and adhere to their requirement for consent. (https://standards.gdc-uk.org/)

Examination tips:

• Be completely familiar with the GDC standards document

• Be completely familiar with the indications, side effects and complications of a dental extraction, a surgical dental extraction and a biopsy

• Practise these with a colleague and ensure a tutor witnesses you and get feedback

• In an examination include every possible complication, starting with the most common, even though it is not likely to occur except in negligence such as numbing the mental nerve during a forceps extraction. (Fractures of the mandible are extremely rare but mention the possibility in an examination).

04 Assessment for Extractions

Assessment of teeth for dental extraction will become instinctive with some experience but initially it should be approached in a logical systematic manner. You should be able to justify each stage in that process in an examination.

Most patients who are being considered for dental extractions will have had pain as a presenting complaint. You should therefore become familiar with taking a pain history. You may find it useful as a beginner to be guided by the SOCRATES mnemonic which we have reproduced.

After the history the patient should be examined. Look for facial swelling which might be firm and/or warm if the patient has an established abscess or may be soft in an early abscess caused by soft tissue oedema. Look for limitation of mouth opening, intra-oral swelling, discharging pus from a sinus or periodontal ligament, tooth loosening including a small degree of lateral mobility, tenderness of the teeth with light pressure or on percussion with an instrument and obviously dental caries and periodontal disease. If a tooth is tender to percussion it suggests that pulpitis has progressed to an apical periodontitis or a dental abscess. If the tooth is slightly more mobile than its neighbours it may be so because of bone resorption caused by periapical infection.

Radiographic examination is nearly always required. If the cause of the pain is unclear pulp sensitivity testing can be used but it has to be interpreted with caution; it can give conflicting evidence but this does not mean it shouldn't be done, rather it should be interpreted with the other examination findings and the history

Periapical periodontitis often progresses to an acute periapical abscess; it may also progress to a chronic abscess which is painless because the pus is draining through a sinus. The former may show a widened periodontal membrane on a radiograph and

---

SOCRATES pain history mnemonic

- **S**ite: where the pain is felt and where is the area it is, or has been, most intense

- **O**nset: when did the pain start and stop (if it has)

- **C**haracter: describe the nature of the pain: is it sharp (as might be associated with a pulpitis), dull (which may be associated with an apical periodontist or muscular pain from masseter or temporalis)

- **R**adiation: does the pain radiate away from the main area; dental pain can radiate from mandible to maxilla or vice versa but never from side to side

- **A**ssociations: any other symptoms related to the history such as swelling, tooth loosening (which might suggest an abscess) or limitation of mouth opening (which might suggest severe infection or internal derangement of the temporomandibular joint)

- **T**ime: Length of symptoms

- **E**xacerbating or relieving factors: such as temperature change from hot or cold food or drinks which might suggest pulpal pain or pressure from chewing which might suggest an apical periodontitis or abscess.

- **S**everity: ask the patient to describe how severe the pain is

---

then later a more defined radiolucency in the bone. However the resorption of mineralised bone which causes the radiolucency will take some time and the radiographic appearance may lag behind the clinical condition by up to 10 days so it is possible for there to be no bony lesion seen on X-ray in the acute situation.

Recommendations should be made to the patient in conjunction with their general medical condition and their general dental state taking into account history of previous dental treatment history and future intentions.

The first thing to consider is the diagnosis and reason for a proposed extraction and a consideration as to why the tooth is not being restored. In some cases a tooth may be diseased with caries, periodontal disease, trauma damage, be non-functional, over erupted or unaesthetic but no treatment at all is to be carried out. This must be considered and the reason justified.

There are several relative contra indications to extraction where it may be desirable to attempt to restore teeth where a long term restorative prognosis may be poor. These include medical conditions such as temporary immunosuppression from chemotherapy and acute illness to local problems such as medication related jaw necrosis and osteonecrosis caused by local radiotherapy (see chapter 02). Some patients may have severe anxiety; this must be addressed (chapter 15).

We do not consider acute infection to be a justified contraindication to extraction with local anaesthetic. Whereas acute inflammation may decrease the effectiveness of local anaesthetic this can be countered by supplementing the usual local injections with intra-ligamentary injection. The theoretical risk of spreading the infection with the local anaesthetic is more than outweighed by the benefit of removing the cause of the infection and allowing the pus to drain.

Once the decision to extract has been made and any medical considerations attended to (chapter 02) the actual procedure should be planned. There are three alternatives to consider:

1. The extraction is expected to be a simple procedure easily accomplished with dental elevators, luxators and/or extraction

Reasons for extracting

- Caries
- Loosened by periodontal disease
- Pain from pulpitis
- Pain from apical periodontitis
- Non vital
- Chronic infection from diseased pulp
- Chronic infection from periodontal disease
- Acute abscess
- Non-functioning and over erupted
- Ectopic position and compromising oral hygiene leading to caries in an adjacent tooth
- Fractured or traumatising soft tissue
- Non-functional and interfering with a proposed prosthesis
- Unaesthetic
- Poor prognosis teeth in area of planned radiotherapy, before bisphosphonate treatment or chemotherapy
- Involvement in a cyst (chapter 20)
- Impacted → pericoronits

Reasons for not restoring

- Patient's wish
- Severe acute abscess
- Unrestorable caries extending sub-gingivally
- Severe periodontal disease
- Non vital curved roots which compromise endodontics
- Non-functional

forceps. In this case the appropriate forceps and elevators are chosen and placed with some sterile swabs on a sterile surface for the dental surgeon to use.

Relative contra-indications to dental extraction

- Acute illness (temporary)
- Bone necrosis (usually bisphosphonates or local radiotherapy)
- Temporary immunosuppression (chemotherapy)
- Risk of jaw fracture
- Tooth close to inferior dental nerve (see chapter 10)

Indicators of simple extraction:

- Periodontal disease
- Short roots
- Single roots
- Conical roots (upper central and lower second premolar)
- Chronic infection

Indicators of Difficult Extraction

- Healthy periodontium
- Long roots
- Divergent roots
- Non vital tooth
- Gross caries (particularly into root)
- Dense bone (some racial groups, particularly Afro-Caribbean))
- Difficult access (e.g. in-standing lower second premolars)
- Bulbous roots

Indicators of definite surgical extraction

- Unerupted tooth
- Bony impaction
- Associated pathology (e.g. cyst)

2. The extraction may be awkward and although a simple extraction is expected there is a distinct possibility that the tooth will break unfavourably during the process and a 'surgical' with elevating of a mucoperiosteal flaps with bone removal or tooth division with a bur will be needed.

3. There is little or no chance that the proposed extraction can be accomplished without a 'surgical' procedure.

In the second case above we often seen the attempted extraction fail and then a nurse is asked to prepare a surgical instrument set and drill, with its irrigation, before proceeding. During the time this takes the patient sits in the dental chair biting on a surgical swab with an impeding sense of doom in the certain knowledge that things have not progressed as intended and becoming even more anxious as a result.

In this case we would counsel that it is better to prepare for a surgical procedure from the outset and tell the patient that the raising of a flap and some drilling may be necessary as it is not really a big deal and certainly less that prolonging a futile attempt with elevators which is always more traumatic for the patient. This is particularly appropriate to first molars which have long roots, have extensive caries and where there is a sound periodontium. The raising of a flap, removal of some bone and division of the roots with a bur prior to elevation will usually result in a shorter and less

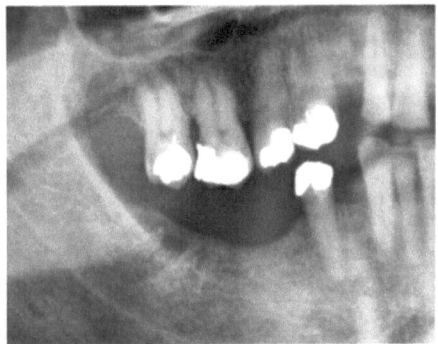

Here the first molar has been unopposed for some time and is over erupted facilitating forceps extraction

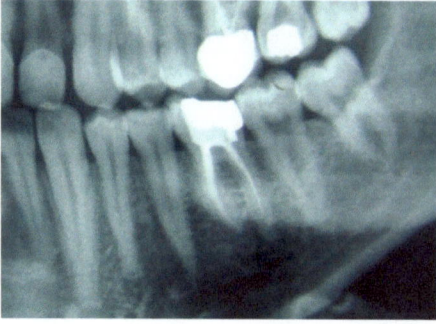

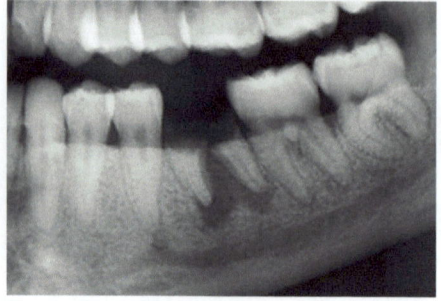

Extensive chronic periapical infection should make for a simple extraction with Warwick James or Cryer's elevators

Everything mitigates against an easy extraction with this lower first molar. It is non vital, root filled, has long roots with one curved and the crown is mostly restoration. Here we would recommend that a surgical procedure with bone removal and division of the tooth is planned from the outset.

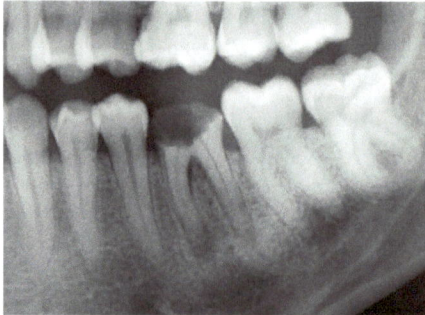

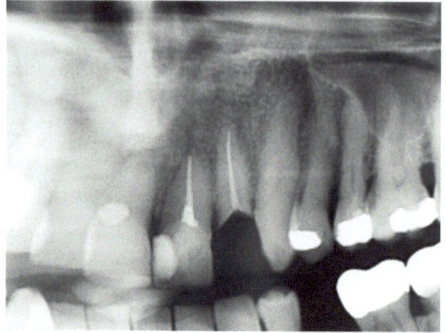

This unrestorable upper canine is non vital, root filled, has a long root (as they do) and there is not much to grip with forceps. A surgical procedure will be needed - difficult.

The reasonable periodontal condition, long roots and non vital nature of the tooth are unfavourable for easy extraction. However the chronic apical infection may have loosened the roots which may split with a Coupland's elevator and be amenable to elevation with Cryer's elevators and root forceps.

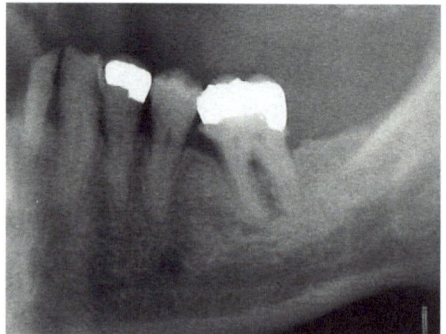

The periodontal disease around this first molar has involved the furcation. The tooth should easily be dispatched with lower molar forceps.

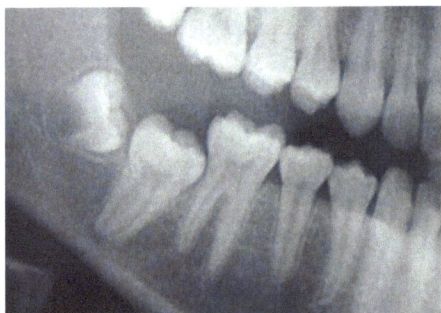

Removal of the second molar will produce a small risk of jaw fracture. This must be discussed with the patient; if the tooth is asymptomatic there is little justification to proceeding.

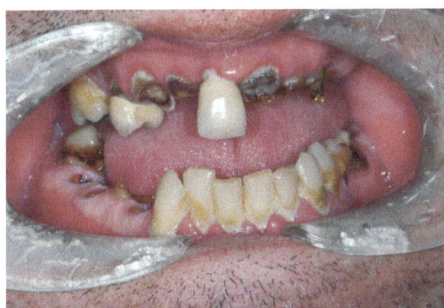

These multiple carious teeth should be straightforward to remove with forceps after loosening them with elevators as the alveolar bone will be resorbed by periodontal disease and infections

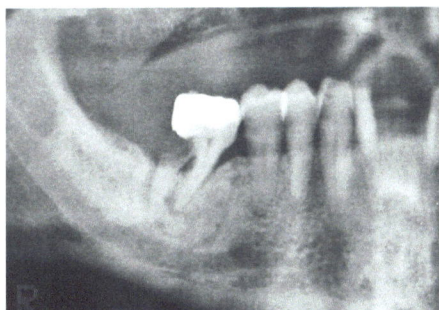

Easy or not?

23

05 Elevators and Forceps

Before attempting a dental extraction you should know what instruments you will need to use and how to hold them and use them safely.

There is a vast variety of elevators and forceps which may be used; many dentists swear by their favourite forceps or elevator which has served them well over the years.

Luxators can be used for cutting periodontal ligament fibres and enlarging the socket by applying apical pressure and a slight wiggling movement. They are best used for single rooted teeth or those with convergent roots.

We will describe the basic instruments needed to accomplish the task you should be able to carry out all dental extractions with the instruments below.

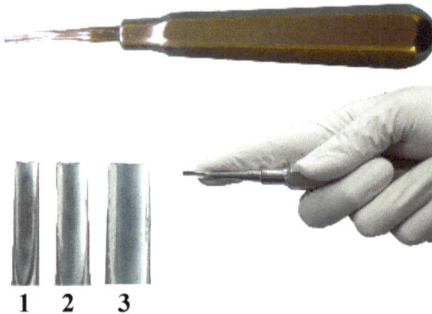

Elevators in order of frequency of use:
- Couplands: 1,2 and 3
- Warwick James: left, right and straight
- Cryers: left and right

Extraction forceps:
- Premolar forceps: upper and lower + narrow version for roots
- Lower molar forceps
- Upper molar forceps: left and right
- Upper straight forceps
- Cowhorns (lower molars)

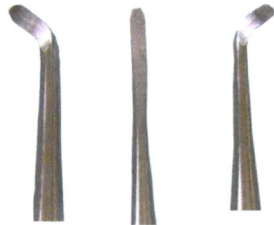

Warwick James come as a trio. Left, straight and right. The straight can penetrate small spaces between bone and tooth to start movement before elevation with a Coupland's and the curved can be used to elevate superficial retained roots.

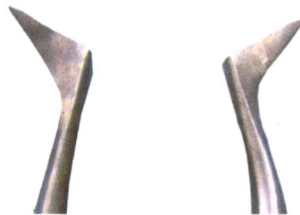

1 2 3

Coupland's elevators are the most frequently used, both for loosening teeth before applying forceps and for elevating tooth fragments and roots if they break during extraction or after bone removal in a surgical extraction. They come in sets of three of increasing size. They are used with a twisting movement between bone and tooth starting with the smallest (No. 1) and increasing to 2 & 3 once movement is achieved. Never use them like a tyre lever; you will probably break the tooth and possibly the jaw. They are also useful for splitting a tooth. Note the fore finger position so that if you slip it won't penetrate far.

Cryer's elevators also come as a pair. The tip is placed between bone and tooth and twisted. The tip can be placed down the socket of a removed root to elevate its neighbour.

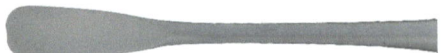

Luxators vary from 2 mm's to 5 mm's width and can have straight or slightly curved handles. They are sharp and can be pushed down a periodontal membrane to loosen a tooth or root.

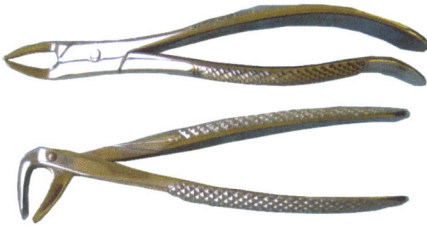

The most useful instruments for dental extraction are the premolar forceps (sometimes called 'universals'), upper and lower. They are the only ones needed to lift teeth out during surgical extractions after removing bone and loosening with elevators.

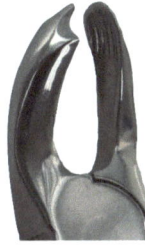

Upper molar forceps. The beaks engage with the tip in the furcation between the two roots on the buccal side and the opposite blade on the single palatal root. Therefore it is necessary to have separate forceps for upper left and right.

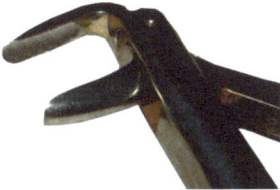

The sharp end of the beaks should be firmly pressed down the periodontal membrane, breaking it down in the process to engage the root. There is a narrow version of these forceps specifically to remove retained roots. They are referred to as upper or lower root forceps.

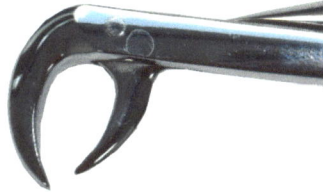

Cowhorns, sometimes used for lower molars. The beaks fit between the roots and are suitable for teeth already loosened. Their advantage is that if the tooth fractures it will probably separate the roots making them susceptible to elevation

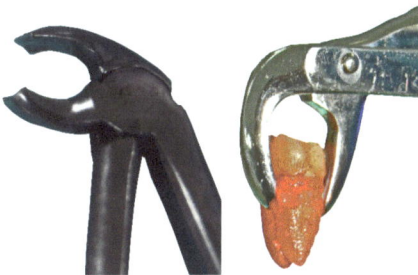

Lower molar forceps. The tip engages the furcation so that the blade will grip both the mesial and distal roots firmly. When using forceps gently force the beaks down the periodontal membrane so they engage with the roots rather than the crown before attempting movement.

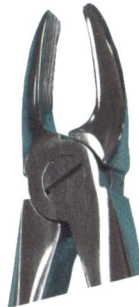

Upper straight handled forceps have blades the same as premolar forceps but having a straight handle gives a better mechanical advantage for removing upper incisors and canines. There is a narrower version for removing roots.

06 Preparing for a Simple Extraction

We recommend that you make yourself familiar with the British Dental Association pamphlet: Infection Control - England, which explains most of what you need to know about cross infection control in concise terms (Appendix 3). You should become familiar with the following procedures needed before a simple dental extraction.

When we anticipate an extraction will be possible without a 'surgical' procedure i.e. without raising a mucoperiosteal flap, division of the tooth or removal of bone (see chapter 08) then we use a simple tray of instruments with a few essentials on it and add the extraction forceps and elevators appropriate for the tooth being removed; these are normally separately wrapped in individual sterile pouches.

Where a surgical procedure is contemplated it is usual to use a surgical tray containing all the instruments we are likely to use; in addition a sterile surgical hand piece with a bur will be needed and the connection to the motor will be covered in a clear barrier sleeve.

You should understand that we are not operating in a sterile environment. The mouth is teeming with bacteria which inevitably will contaminate our surgical wounds whatever we do. Fortunately the jaws are very resistant to infection. If an orthopaedic surgeon made a hole in a femur the size of an extraction socket and contaminated it with saliva osteomyelitis would almost certainly result.

By these procedures we are attempting to prevent infection from one patient to another, from any patient to ourselves and from ourselves to a patient. In addition we are demonstrating a cosmetically clean environment which the patient, and anyone else, can be confident with. In some hospitals you may find that these procedures are undertaken with the operator wearing full surgical gowns and sterile surgical gloves. We believe we can achieve our objectives wearing Personal Protective Equipment (PPE) - disposable plastic aprons, face masks and examination gloves.

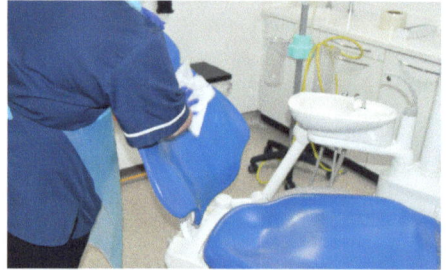

1. The dental chair is cleaned with an alcohol impregnated disinfectant surface wipe

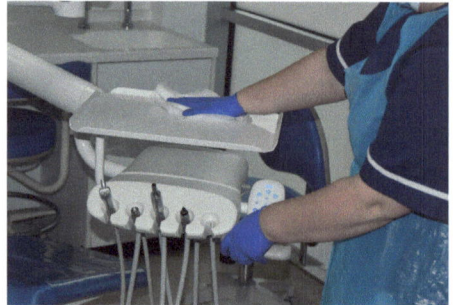

2. Bracket table, light, other parts of the dental unit are similarly cleaned

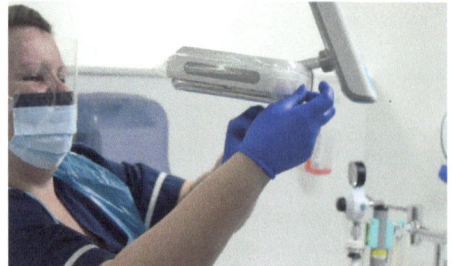

3. A clear barrier film is wrapped around the light handle

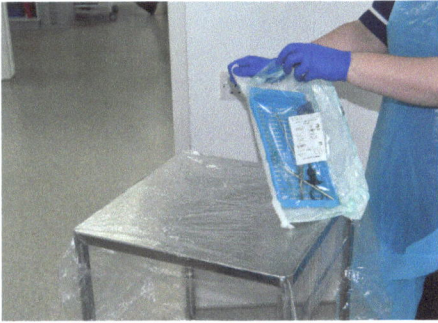

4. The instruments are placed on a surgical trolley which has been cleaned with an alcohol wipe and covered with a barrier film

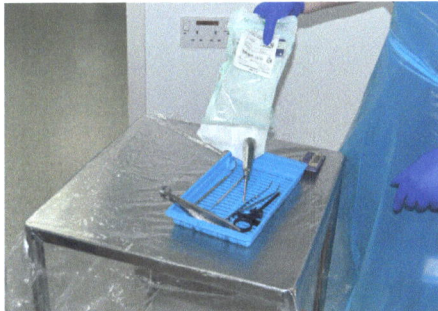

5. A sterile extraction tray has been dropped from its wrapping onto the trolley and for simple extractions other instruments are added from individual packs

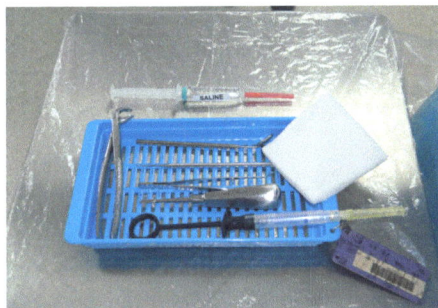

6. Ready to go: tray with probe, college forceps, mouth mirror, extraction forceps. Elevator, aspirating syringe, saline, surgical gauze

Putting on personal protective equipment (PPE)

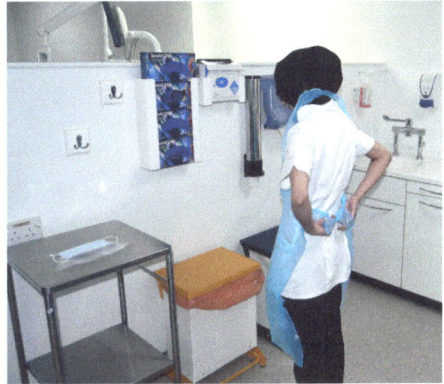

1. Put on protective apron

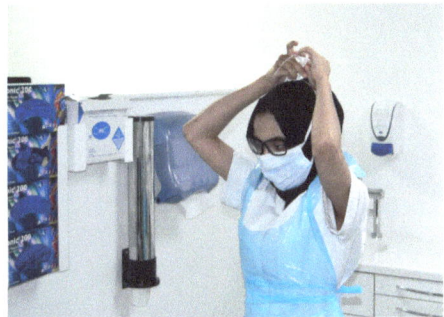

2. Face mask

Washing hands before minor oral surgery
Should only take 15 to 30 seconds

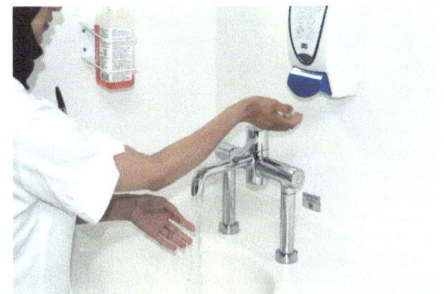

1. Take off rings and watches and ensure bare below elbows, turn on taps and wet hands thoroughly, apply soap enough to cover hands completely

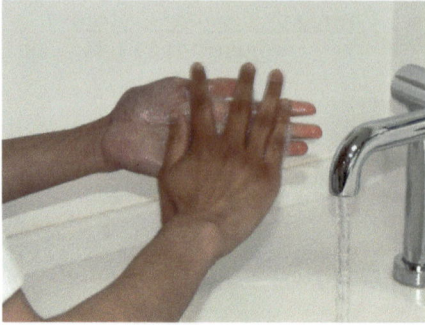

2. Rub palms together to generate a good lather

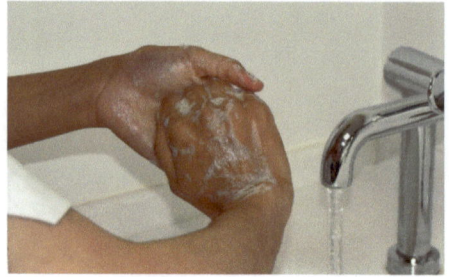

5. Cup hands together to clean back of fingers and nails

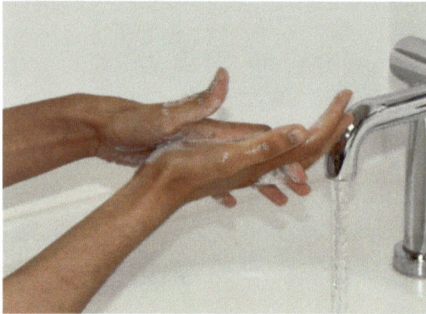

3. Rub palms together with fingers interlocked

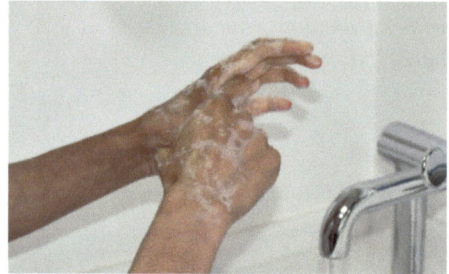

6. Scrub thumbs with a twisting motion, making sure you get into pits

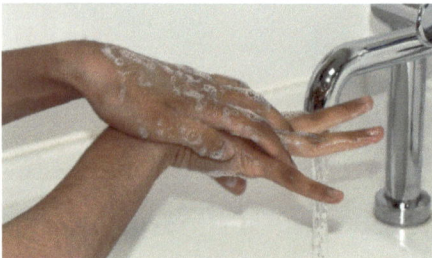

4. Rub the back of each hand with palm of the other with fingers interlocked

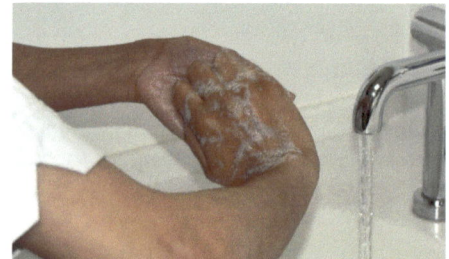

7. Rub the tip of fingers against palm of hands in a circular motion (to clean nails)

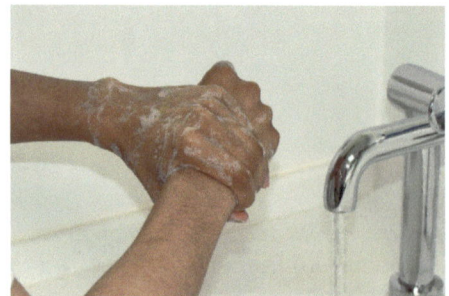

8. Wash the wrists

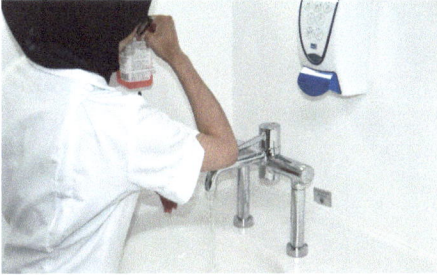

9. Rinse hands thoroughly, turn off taps with elbows, dry hands with a single use towel

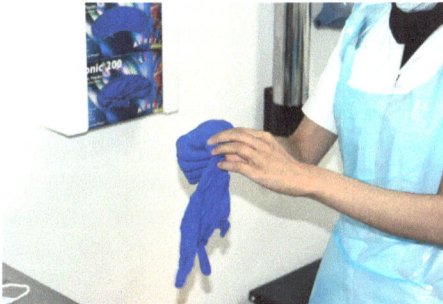

10. Protective gloves. Note that in some hospital departments it may be the convention to use sterile surgical gloves

Equipment disposal after the procedure

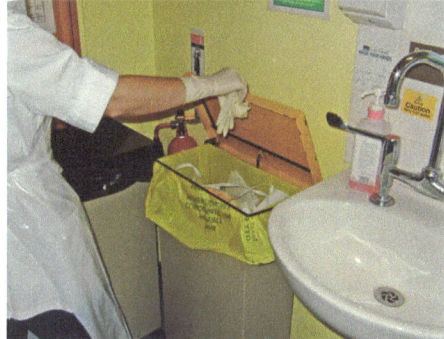

Not sharp clinical waste: swabs, PPE anything potentially contaminated with blood or saliva goes into a yellow clinical waste bag. Uncontaminated waste goes into a domestic waste bag

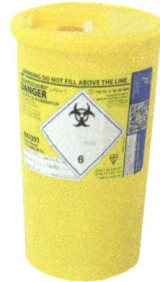

Sharps: needles, sutures tooth fragments go into a sharps box. But not teeth with amalgam, these should be disposed of separately

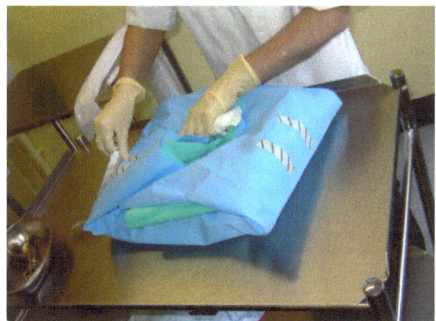

Instruments are re wrapped as they came and placed in a secure trolley to return to sterile supply

07 Simple Extractions - Technique

Once the decision for an extraction has been made, the patient has given their consent in writing as well as verbally, they have been made aware of potential side effects and complications, you are ready to start.

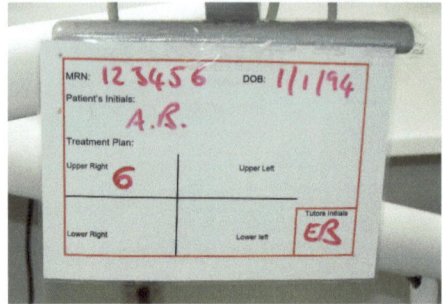

In the student's clinic we attach a chart to the chair to help avoid mistakes

You must select which forceps and elevators or luxators you will need and have a surgical set of instruments available should your assessment indicate that this may be necessary. We repeat that it is much slicker to have this open and ready to go with drill set up and primed if this is likely to be needed.

The patient should be seated comfortably in the chair with a bib and you must don personal protective equipment - eye protection (safety glasses), mask, apron and gloves. It is useful to have a written record of the tooth that is to be removed visible. This may be the patient's clinical notes (open at the relevant page), the consent form or as in our extraction clinic a chart attached to the chair, as shown below.

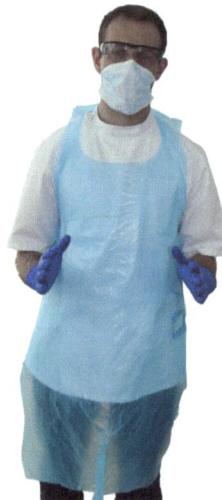

Dressed for action in personal protective equipment (PPE) - disposable apron, mask, eye protection and disposable examination gloves. We don't think a sterile theatre gown and sterile gloves are necessary

We will now go through our recommended technique for removing individual teeth; the anatomical diagrams all relate to teeth on the patient's right hand

---

Before starting check:

1. The patient's identity

2. Confirm the procedure to be carried out

3. Confirm they know the side effects and possible complications

4. Consent has been confirmed on a consent form

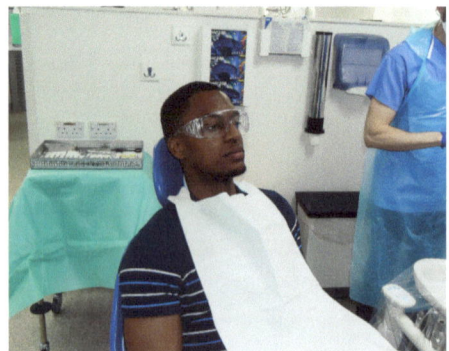

Patient should be comfortably seated wearing a protective bib and eye protection

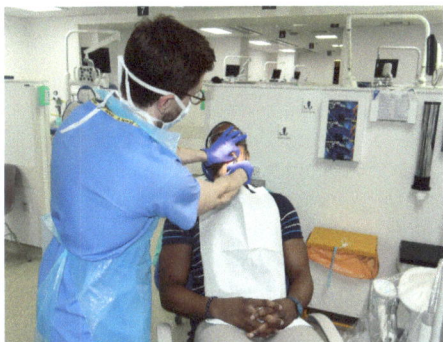

When using forceps stand firmly on two feet with a straight back

For the removal of any teeth with forceps the primary movement is apical pressure with the beaks of the forceps forced up the periodontal ligament and engaging the root of the tooth with a tight grip. The secondary movements for each individual tooth will differ according to the root morphology; these we will describe. While using forceps, elevators or luxators always support the alveolus or mandible with your non-dominant hand.

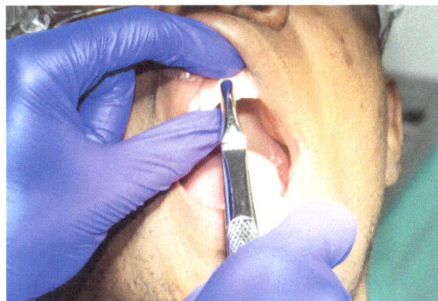

Upper Incisors

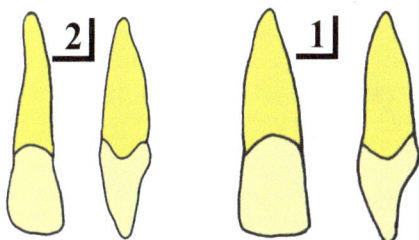

The upper central incisor has a longish root but it is very nearly conical making it usually easy to remove by rotation with the forceps. The lateral incisor root is slightly shorter but the root is wider antero-posteriorly than from a labial aspect, making it less easily rotated.

If several teeth in a row are to be removed, they may be loosened by rotating successively larger Coupland's elevators between them, alternatively luxators may be used, they are useful with single straight rooted teeth. Do not attempt elevation if one tooth only is to be extracted as you may

Hand position for removing upper central incisors. For this and all other extractions you should use your non-dominant hand to steady the alveolus or mandible

damage the adjacent ones; the risk may be reduced if using a luxator. Both central and lateral incisors may be removed fairly easily with upper straight forceps. Engage the root with the end of the beaks and in the case of the central use a rotating motion only. For the lateral loosen with a combination of rotation and labial movement. If there is caries extending well into the root then use root forceps.

Upper Canine

The upper canine is the tooth with the longest roots and wider in the buccal-palatal plane than anterior-posterior, meaning it is not very susceptible to rotation. Again we advise caution in using elevators as it is easy to damage the adjacent teeth although the risk is less with luxators. Some considerable controlled force is usually necessary with upper straight forceps to dislodge the tooth initially with a buccal movement and then some rotation to enlarge the socket. If the root is carious the use of root forceps is unlikely to give sufficient purchase to dislodge it and surgical removal of bone with a bur and elevation from above may been needed.

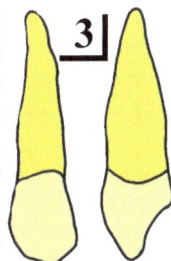

Upper Premolars

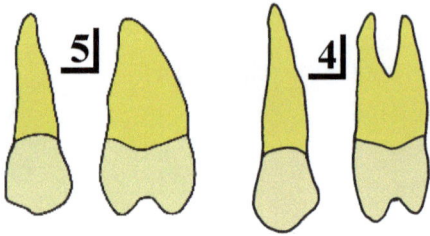

The premolars are the first teeth (as you progress distally) that you can become confident that, with skill, you can use a Coupland's elevator to loosen the teeth before applying forceps without harming their neighbour.

Upper premolar forceps should be used to apply slight buccal pressure before wiggling the tooth around to expand the bony socket before bending it buccally to extract.

Upper 5s are single rooted and are often amenable to rotation but the upper 4 is more problematical because it has two roots and sometimes these can be quite fine; the palatal one may snap off. If most of the root is retained it may be possible to elevate it from the buccal root socket with a curved Warwick James or Cryer's elevator. It may yield to the application of a fine luxator down the side of the retained fragment. If less than half of the root is retained then a decision should be made as to whether to carry out a surgical procedure and remove bone to retrieve it. In most cases it may be better to leave it as the root will most likely remain asymptomatic for ever. The patient should be warned that the root may work its way to the surface in which case it will be easily removed with an elevator. The decision should be made in accordance with the patient's dental and medical condition. If a bridge or an implant is intended it will probably be better removed.

Upper First and Second Molars

The upper first and second molars have two buccal roots (which may be quite delicate and break easily) and one palatal root which is much longer and and broader. The buccal roots are usually close to the maxillary antrum and rarely an oro-antral communication may result from their removal (see chapter 13).

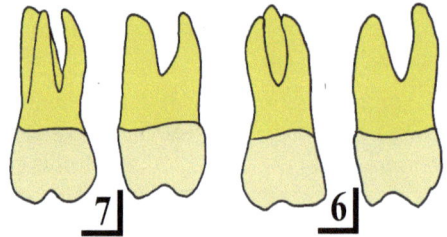

If one or both of the buccal roots are very carious then you may well be better off carrying out a surgical approach from the beginning and splitting the crown vertically and elevating the mesio-buccal root first and hope that the palatal root elevates with the remainder of the crown with the distal root. It usually does.

Normally you should loosen the tooth with elevators starting with a straight Warwick James and then successively larger Coupland's before removing the tooth buccally with molar forceps.

If the roots break off you may attempt to elevate them downwards with curved Warwick James or Cryer's elevators but be aware that if careless you can push them into the maxillary antrum, especially if pushing upwards forcefully with root forceps.

Upper Third Molars

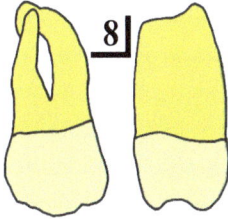

The upper third molar has variable root morphology; it may have two roots or they may be fused into one. The tooth is often in an ectopic position usually inclined bucco-distally. The roots are usually shortish so it may be easily elevated distally with curved Warwick James or Cryer's elevators. However, if it is within the dental arch and not bucco-distally inclined it should be removed with upper premolar forceps which usually dispatch the tooth swiftly. Bayonet forceps designed to cope with the more difficult access at the back of the mouth give inferior grip on the tooth. It is very rare for a surgical procedure to be needed or an oro-antral communication to arise from an upper 8 extraction.

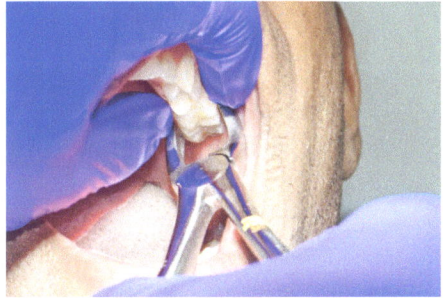

Hand position for removal of upper right molar. Upper 1st and 2nd molars have 3 roots. Upper 3rd molars usually have short roots and are more easily removed, but beware that elevating them distally may fracture the maxillary tuberosity

NB: *Remember to take care of your back. Do not twist or bend in order to reach the patient. Use the controls on the chair in order to achieve a comfortable position. Keep your back straight whilst performing exodontia*

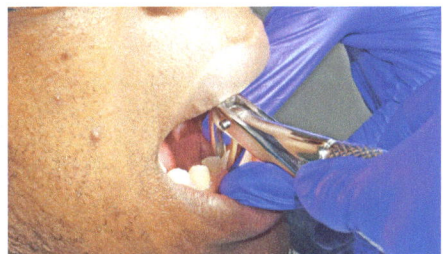

Hand position for removal of upper left molars. The forceps are used after the tooth has been loosened by expanding the socket using elevators. Further loosen the tooth with a slight rotating motion while twisting it buccally

Lower Incisors

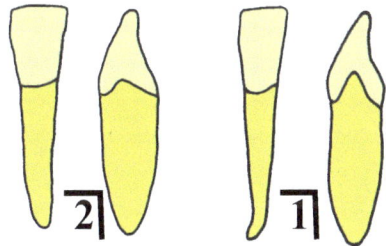

The lower incisors are usually easy to remove. As with the upper incisors we suggest you do not attempt to loosen with an elevator unless you are extracting several together as it is easy to damage the adjacent teeth. They are usually too narrow to apply lower premolar forceps so we suggest that you use the narrower lower root forceps with a slight buccal movement followed by some rotation and gentle wiggling to enlarge the socket before taking the tooth out buccally.

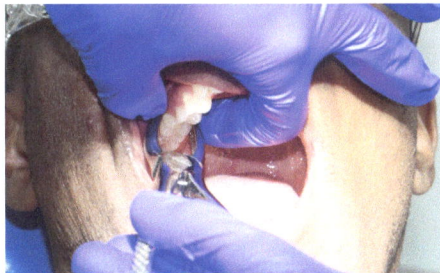

Removing lower incisors

Lower Canines

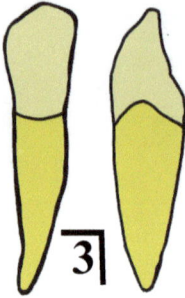

The lower canine has long roots but not as unfavourable as the upper and is more susceptible to rotation. Again we advise against using elevators as to do so risks damage to the adjacent incisor or premolar. Use lower premolar forceps and start with some slight rotation followed by buccal movement, gradually increasing the movement as the socket enlarges before removing it buccally.

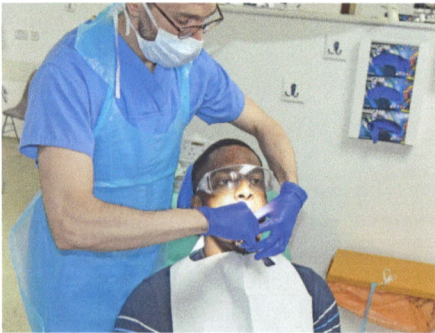

For lower incisors and canines stand just behind the patient for right hand side teeth and in front for left. Use a combination of buccal and rotational movements

Lower First and Second Premolars

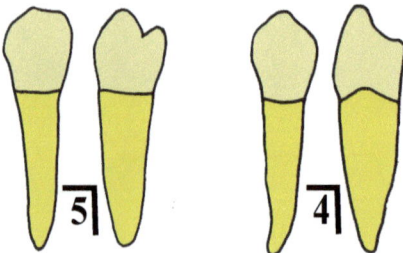

The lower first premolar may be loosened slightly with a straight Warwick James elevator followed by a No.1 Coupland's if necessary and then dispatched with lower premolar forceps. The second premolar has a conical root and is easily removed with forceps using a rotating movement.

Lower First and Second Molars

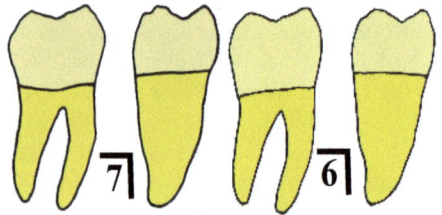

Lower first and second molars can be difficult to remove as they have two roots which are often quite long and slender and may be curved unfavourably. The lower 6 is the first to erupt and you may be presented with young patients with advanced caries and a healthy periodontium. In this circumstance it is often simpler, quicker and less traumatic to undertake a surgical procedure from the outset and after removing buccal bone split the tooth vertically and elevate the roots separately rather than risk them breaking off low down. It may be possible to use cowhorn forceps which engage below the furcation, they may split the roots apart making them easier to remove individually.

If attempting a non-surgical extraction start by loosening with a straight Warwick James and then Coupland's before using molar forceps to take the tooth buccally after expanding the socket in a figure of eight movement.

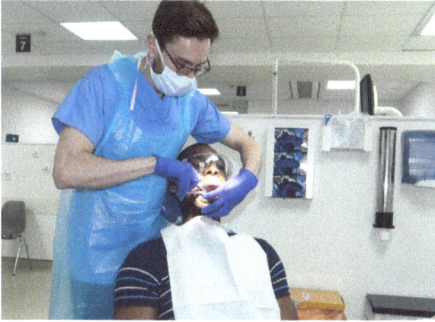

For lower right teeth stand behind the patient thus

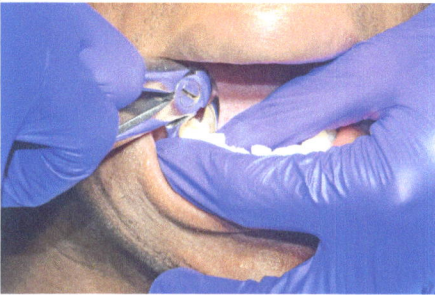

Hand positions lower molars. RHS above LHS below

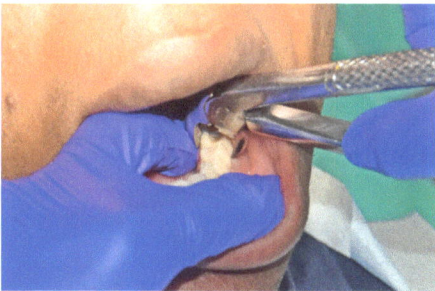

We will discuss lower third molar removal in chapter 10

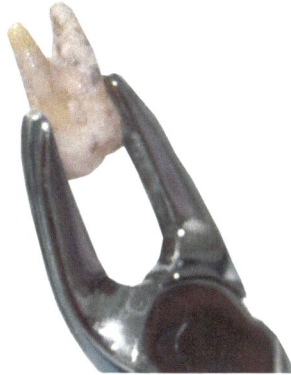

The primary movement for all exodontia with forceps is always apical pressure. This should be accomplished with the beaks engaging the roots as shown

Summary of secondary movements for exodontia upper teeth
(The primary movement is always apical pressure)

Tooth	Movement
Central Incisor	Rotate
Lateral Incisor	Rotate & buccal
Canine	Rotate
1st & 2nd premolars	Buccal
1st & 2nd molars	Buccal
3rd molar	Buccal/distal elevation

Lower teeth

Tooth	Movement
Incisors	Bucco-lingual
Canine	Rotate
1st premolar	Rotate and buccal
2nd premolar	Rotate
1st & 2nd molars	Figure of 8 followed by buccal
3rd molar	Lingual (forceps not recommended)

Operator and Chair Positions for exodontia.

Right handed operator

UR Quadrant	UL Quadrant
Patient position: Chair reclined to 45° and pt's mouth at shoulder height	Patient position: Chair reclined to 45° and pt's mouth at shoulder height
Operator position: Stand in front of pt on their right side	Operator position: Stand in front of pt on their right side
LR Quadrant	**LL Quadrant**
Patient position: Chair reclined slightly and pt's mouth at elbow height	Patient position: Chair reclined slightly and pt's mouth at elbow height
Operator position: Stand behind patient on right side	Operator position: Stand in front of patient on their right side/standing on left is also acceptable

Left handed operator

UR Quadrant	UL Quadrant
Patient position: Chair reclined to 45° and pt's mouth at shoulder height	Patient position: Chair reclined to 45° and pt's mouth at shoulder height
Operator position: Stand in front of pt on their left side. Acceptable to stand on right side as well	Operator position: Stand in front of pt on their left side.
LR Quadrant	**LL Quadrant**
Patient position: Chair reclined slightly and pt's mouth at elbow height	Patient position: Chair reclined slightly and pt's mouth at elbow height
Operator position: Stand in front on right side	Operator position: Stand behind and slightly to the left

08 Principles of Surgical Extraction

Many diseased teeth will not submit to a simple extraction with forceps and/or elevators and will need bone removal to facilitate their removal. In some cases an attempt at forceps and elevator extraction will fail and a surgical procedure will found to be necessary. However with proper assessment this can usually be predicted. With experience this becomes intuitive but those with less experience and, particularly for examinations, each case must be assessed in stages. It is quicker and less unpleasant for the patient to have a planned surgical procedure than a prolonged attempt with forceps and elevators which later becomes a surgical.

It will be necessary to have an assistant. The setting up process will involve you both with the assistant opening the instrument tray touching only the outside of the wrapping and opening the extras such as blade, bur, swabs and sutures and letting them drop onto the open trays.

We have listed the factors to consider when contemplating a surgical procedure below.

A flap of mucosa and periosteum must be raised to get access to the bone and roots. The flap design should be planned to give adequate access and have a good blood supply. The flap should avoid the lingual nerve, the mental nerve and the

---

> ### *Principles of flap design*
> - Margin on sound bone
> - Margin away from area of bone removal
> - Wide based flap to facilitate blood supply from distally
> - Should include interdental papilla for suturing
> ### *Should avoid:*
> - Lingual nerve
> - Mental nerve
> - Canine eminence

---

canine eminence. The interdental papilla at the edge of the flap (which is easy to suture) should be intact and the edge of the flap should be on healthy bone away from the mental nerve and the area of bone and tooth removal; this makes it less likely to break down. In nearly all cases this means a two sided flap with the upper margin in the periodontal membranes of the teeth and includes the interdental papillae and the other margin anterior as the blood supply mostly comes from distally. The anterior margin should extend down from the attached gingivae just into the reflected mucosa. A flap which is too small will compromise visibility of the operation site,

---

> ### *Factors mitigating against a forceps/elevator simple extraction*
> - Multiple divergent roots
> - Non vital tooth therefore brittle
> - Very carious crown
> - Carious root
> - Healthy periodontium
> - Some racial groups have very dense bone, particularly Afro-Caribbean

---

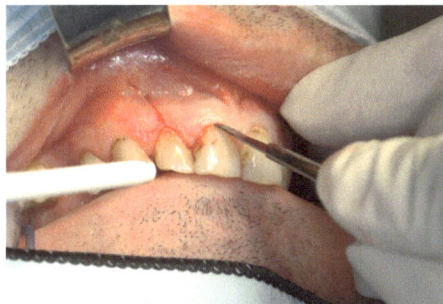

The incision for a flap (in this case for a maxillary cyst) shows the vertical incision only just into the reflected mucosa and the interdental papilla included in the flap for ease of suturing

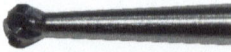

Round bur

Fissure bur

will prolong the procedure and will be more likely to break down afterwards.

Bone removal is accomplished with a hand piece and disposable stainless steel burs. Usually a rounded headed bur and a fissure bur are used. These are irrigated with sterile saline which cools the bur and washes the bone, tooth fragments and blood away, facilitating good vision.

Bone removal serves three purposes and the procedure is planned with these in mind. It allows access to the roots of the tooth that needs extraction, it creates space for an elevator to be fitted between root and bone, and it creates space for the tooth root to be elevated into on its way out. A bur is also used to divide roots particularly in molar teeth with two or three roots, particularly if divergent.

Once the tooth fragments are loose they are removed with Fickling forceps as are any loose pieces of bone. Sharp or rough parts of the remaining alveolus may be smoothed but any trimming should be quick and minimal; the soft tissue flap should never be trimmed.

Suturing should lightly position the soft tissue flap back into place. Sutures should be the minimum necessary to achieve this and the anterior margin should be sufficiently loose to allow the escape of any subsequent bleeding which would cause bruising and swelling if trapped beneath the flap.

The patient should then bite on a damp surgical swab for 10 minutes and be given verbal instructions on care of the wound, what to do in the event of excessive bleeding and where to get help if necessary. They should be given a written copy of the instructions, some swabs to bite on if there is further bleeding and the first dose of

analgesia so that it has some effect when the numbness wears off. After about 10 minutes if all is well they can go home.

Afterwards the instruments are placed back in the trays which are wrapped and sent back to the sterile supply department. They are not washed by hand but by machine before being repacked and then autoclaved in steam at 134 to 137 °C at 2 bar pressure for 3 to 3½ minutes.

Surgical Extraction of a Lower First Molar

A neatly executed surgical extraction which has been adequately prepared for and planned is less traumatic to the tissue and less unpleasant for the patient than an attempted but failed simple extraction with forceps and elevators alone.

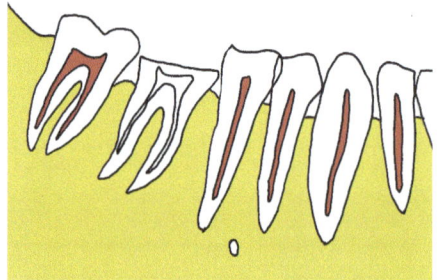

1. Here is a lower first molar which had two long roots, is non vital, has a fractured crown and is surrounded by a healthy periodontium so we are going to remove it surgically

2. After the patient is seated and comfortable the proposed surgery is explained and consent given. Local anaesthesia is administered and a soft tissue flap raised to get access to the bone. and roots

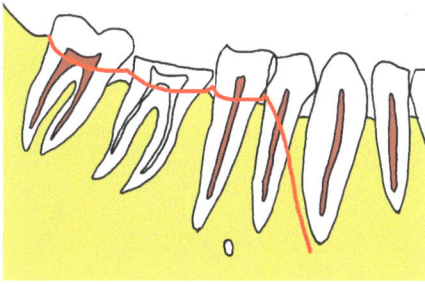

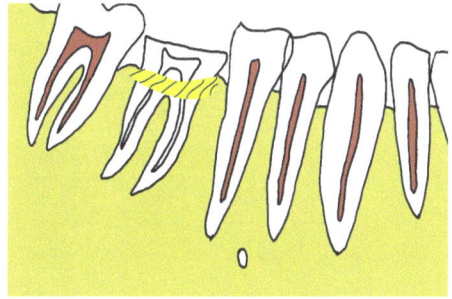

3. Two incisions are made in two movements with the blade pressed firmly though the mucosa and periosteum below it. The first down the periodontal ligament from the distal margin of the seven and forward to include the interdental papilla between the premolars which we are going to suture. The anterior cut extends down and forward so that there is at least one tooth's width of healthy bone between the operation site and edge of the wound. The incision extends off the attached mucosa just into the reflected mucosa but not far as we don't wish to cause excess bleeding or damage the mental

5. The flap is retracted and a gutter of bone removed buccally around the crown just down to the furcation area, here marked in yellow hatched. This is usually accomplished with a round bur

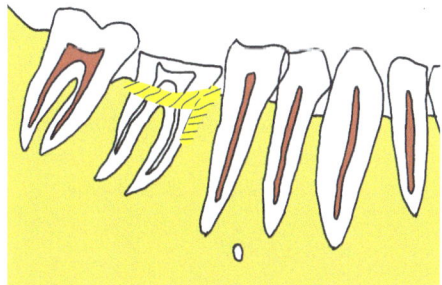

6. Bone is removed mesially of the tooth, usually with a fissure bur to get access down the root and to create space for a Coupland's elevator to be placed

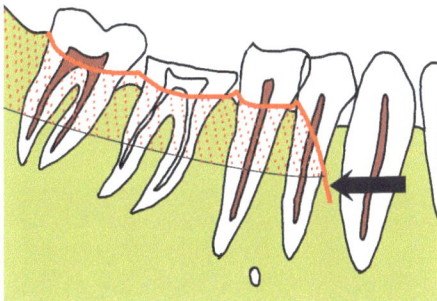

4. The red hatched area represents the attached gingiva where the stratified squamous epithelium is very adherent to the periosteum beneath which itself is firmly attached to the alveolar bone. Attempting to raise the flap from the edge here is likely to cause a tear so start raising the flap from the reflected mucosa just below at the level of the arrow. When the instrument is under the periosteum you can then more easily raise the flap from below

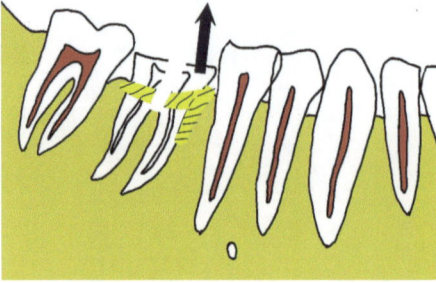

7. *The tooth crown is split vertically down to the furcation with the fissure bur. This allows the two roots to be removed separately and makes space for the mesial root to be elevated into. The mesial root is elevated with the Coupland's elevators starting with number 1. If a good purchase is achieved between root and bone and it will not move then more bone should be removed, not a larger elevator to achieve greater force. The Coupland's 2 and 3 are used when movement with 1 has started. Using a larger elevator to produce more force is likely to fragment the root and make it more difficult*

Examination tips:

▪ Be prepared to give a 'patient' (actor) post operative instructions for a surgical extraction in an OSCE.

▪ Be sure your flap design follows the principles of flap design and be able to justify it.

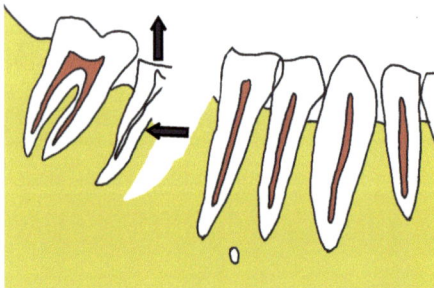

8. *The distal root is elevated with a Cryer's elevator placed down the socket of the mesial root (arrow). Thin bone between the roots will be broken and loose fragments removed. Bone fragments that are not loose can be left for the osteoclasts to deal with. The wound is irrigated lightly and sutured*

09 <u>Instruments and Preparation for a Surgical Extraction</u>

The best way to become familiar with the procedure of surgical extractions is to watch the process yourself. Here we introduce you to the basic instruments found in a minor oral surgery set used for surgical extractions. These are in addition to the forceps and elevators in a previous chapter used where bone removal is not needed. For a surgical it will be necessary to have an assistant and the setting up process will involve you both with the assistant opening the surgical tray where the instruments will be double wrapped, touching only the outside of the wrapping and opening the extras such as blade, bur, swabs and sutures and letting them drop onto the open trays.

<u>Surgical Instuments (not used for simple extractions)</u>

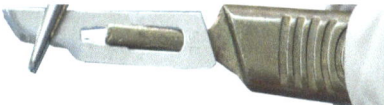

There are various sizes of surgical blade but we always use a round ended size 15a. It should be mounted on the handle using an instrument, not fingers

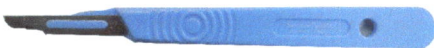

A disposable scalpel and blade are commonly used which reduces the risk of a sharps injury

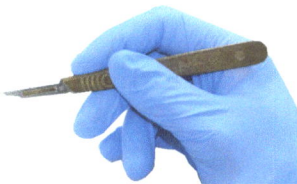

When operating the scalpel should be held with a pen grip and using a finger rest. One cut through mucosa and periosteum should be made with the blade pressed firmly against the bone

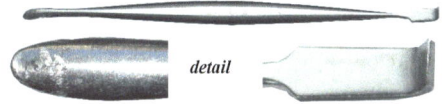

The Howarth's periosteal elevator should be used to raise the flap of mucosa and periosteum together. The periosteum will be firmly adherent to the bone so firm controlled pressure will be needed. The Howarth's may also be used as a retractor.

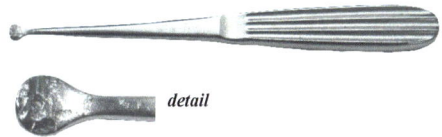

The Ward periosteal elevator has a sharper edge so you may find it easier to get under the mucosa

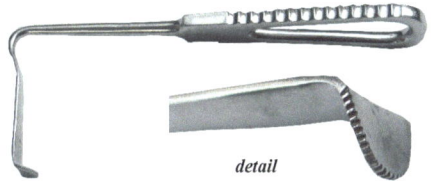

Bowdler Henry rake retractor is used to retract the muco-periosteal flap while drilling

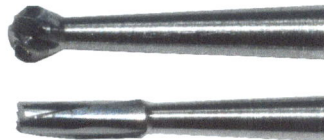

A round ended bur (top) and fissure bur (below) are provided. The round ended bur is useful for removing buccal bone to expose tooth root for access. The fissure bur is most useful for removing bone from mesially or distally of the root to create space to apply an elevator to the root or to elevate the root into. It is also used to divide roots of molars

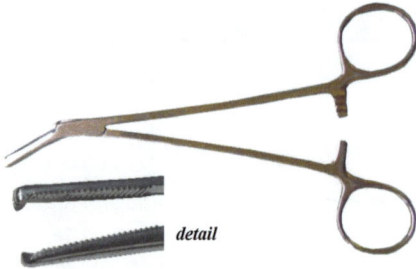

Dental remnants & bone fragments should be removed from the mouth with the Fickling's forceps, not the sucker

Typical Instruments on Minor Oral Surgery Set for Surgical Extractions

- Upper & lower premolar forceps
- Coupland's, Cryer's & Warwick James elevators
- Howarth's and Ward's periosteal elevators
- Bowdler Henry rake retractor
- Kilner cheek retractor
- Fickling forceps
- Needle Holders
- Toothed tissue forceps
- McIndoe scissors

To be added

- Surgical burs, usually one round & one fissure
- Surgical swabs
- Suture
- Surgical blade

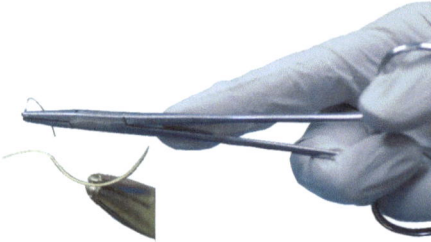

The Crile-Wood needle holders should be used to suture thus. Hold the needle with the end of beaks at 90 degrees

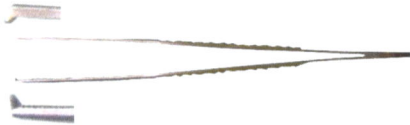

The toothed Gillies forceps are used to hold the flap during suturing

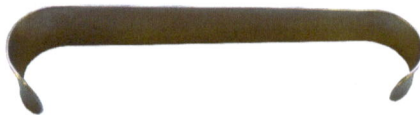

The Kilner cheek retractor can be used to facilitate good vision or protect the angle of the mouth when using the drill

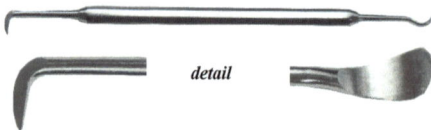

Mitchell's trimmer chiefly used as a curette

Preparation

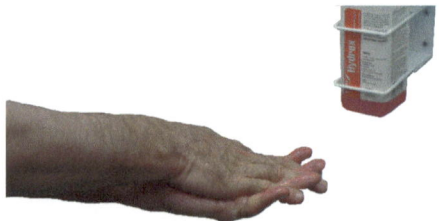

1. Wash Hands

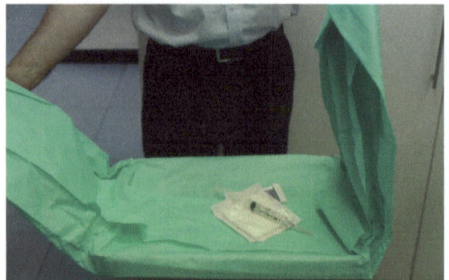

2. Open surgical set on trolley

42

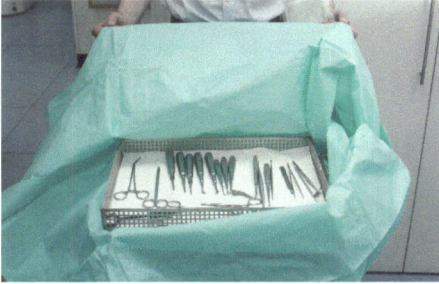

3. Touch only outside of paper

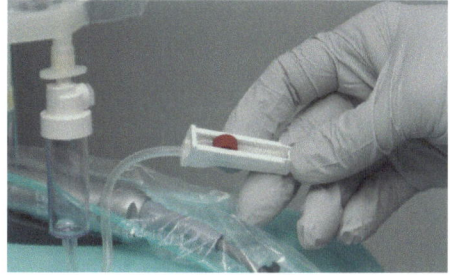

4. Drop sterile swabs, blade, bur & sutures onto the tray by tearing open their packets, touching only the outside

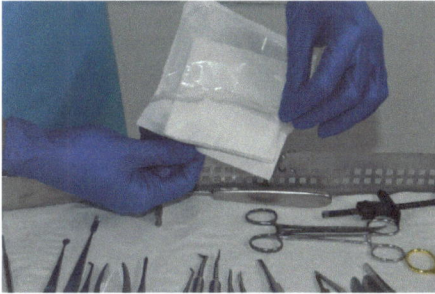

5. Fluid is delivered to the surgical bur from a fluid bag via an intravenous giving set. The handpiece will have been attached to the drill motor by the nurses and covered with a clean plastic sleeve. Push the end of the giving set into port of the fluid bag after removing the protective cap

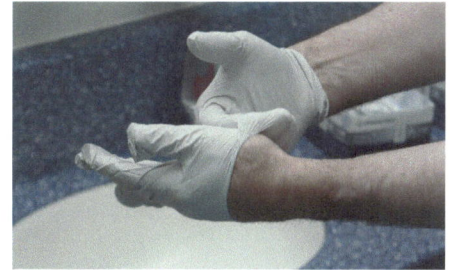

6. Turn on the water at the wheel on the tubing

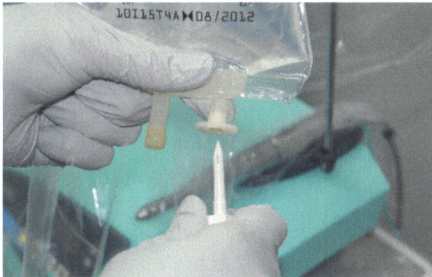

7. Surgeon washes hands & dons gloves. The gloves are clean but not sterile so it is good practice not to touch those parts of the instruments which will contact the surgical wound

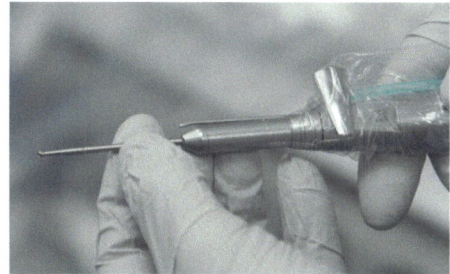

8. Surgeon mounts the surgical bur in the handpiece and checks it is rotating

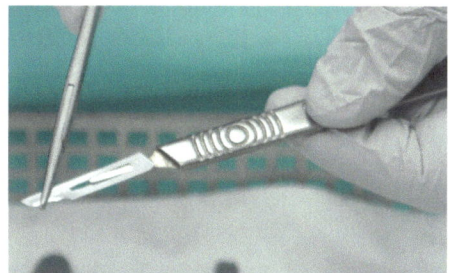

10. Blade is placed on handle with needle holders, not fingers

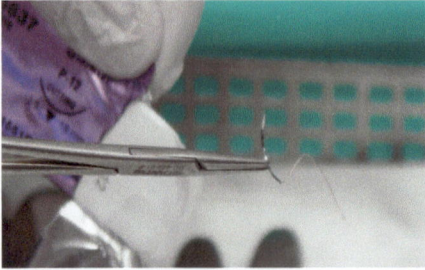

11. Mount the suture needle on the needle holders

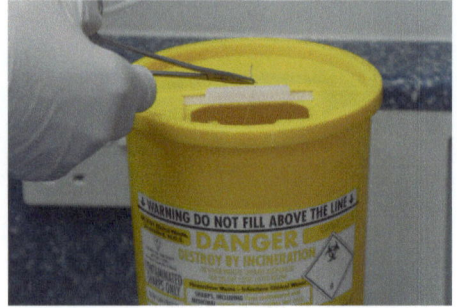

Other sharps: disposable scalpel, sutures, used burs & tooth fragments go in a sharps bin (yellow). Teeth containing amalgam should be disposed of separately

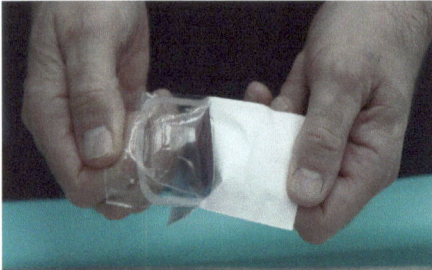

12. You should now be ready to start the surgery. Make sure you wash your hands and wear clean gloves if you have touched anything not sterile such as the fluid bag.

After surgery

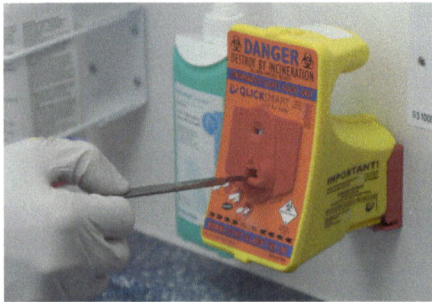

Where a non disposable scalpel is used the blade is disposed of in the 'QLICKsmart' (or similar) blade disposal unit

Instruments for Minor Oral Surgery on tray

1. *Mouth mirror*
2. *Dental probe*
3. *Mitchell's trimmer*
4. *Ward's periosteal elevator*
5. *Howarth's periosteal elevator*
6. *Three Warwick James elevators - right, straight and left*
7. *Two Cryer's elevators - right and left*
8. *Three Coupland's elevators - 1,2 and 3*
9. *Scalpel handle*
10. *Fickling's forceps*
11. *College forceps*
12. *Crile-Wood needle holders*
13. *Toothed tissue forceps*
14. *McIndoe's scissors*
15. *Kilner cheek retractor*
16. *Bowdler Henry rake retractor*
17. *Two mosquito forceps - straight and curved*
18. *Handle for disposable syringe*

Commonly used in minor oral surgery, this suture dissolves fairly quickly and is ideal for dento-alveolar surgery where soft tissue flap support is needed for only a few days. It is fairly brittle and will easily break if you pull too tightly when tying.

10 Impacted Third Molars

You should not be expected to be able to competently remove impacted teeth by the time you qualify as a dental surgeon but you should have a grasp of the main issues, be able to provide first line management for patients presenting with acute problems and if necessary refer them to a colleague with the appropriate experience. Should you get the opportunity to surgically remove impacted teeth under supervision you should seize it as the techniques can be easily learned. Most of the impacted teeth that will present themselves will be impacted third molars or ectopic upper canines.

Mandibular third molars are often impacted because we no longer eat diets which cause sufficient tooth abrasion to allow enough medial drift to make room for them to erupt; usually between the ages of 18 and 24 years.

Third molars will often make their presence known when they are partly erupted and partly covered with soft tissue (the operculum) which can become inflamed when traumatised between the lower and upper teeth. This may lead to mild discomfort on biting or chewing or a full blown infection around the crown (pericoronitis) which can be serious and in the pre-antibiotic era could progress to death from spreading infection down the neck.

> ### NICE indications for third molar removal
>
> - Unrestorable caries
> - Untreatable pulpal or periapical pathology
> - Cellulitis, abscess, osteomyelitis
> - Resorption of the tooth or adjacent teeth
> - Fracture of tooth
> - Cyst or tumour of the follicle
> - Tooth impeding surgery e.g. tumour resection or reconstruction

Pericoronitis is usually managed by grinding or removing the opposing tooth that is traumatising the operculum over the affected tooth. Antibiotics should only be used if their are systemic signs or symptoms. If severe with trismus and infection travelling into and down the neck then hospital admission may be necessary.

Vertically aligned teeth will generally erupt fully but may become impacted in soft tissue if there is insufficient room; this may cause repeated pericoronal infection. Mesially inclined teeth may gradually become vertical after eruption or impact further; they too may lead to pericoronitis, exacerbate oral hygiene and predispose to caries in the distal of the second molar; they

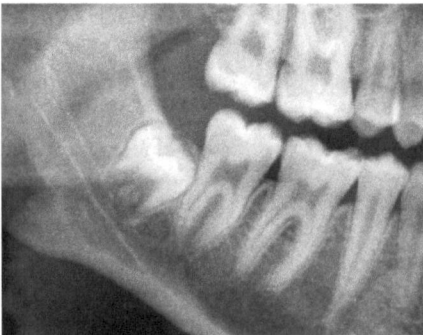

Completely unerupted third molar. This can safely be left alone.

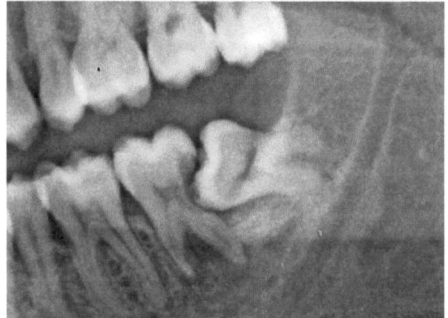

An asymptomatic partly erupted third molar, but it has caused erosion of the adjacent tooth

46

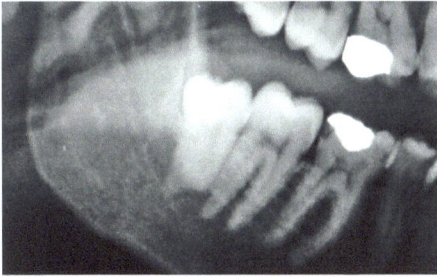

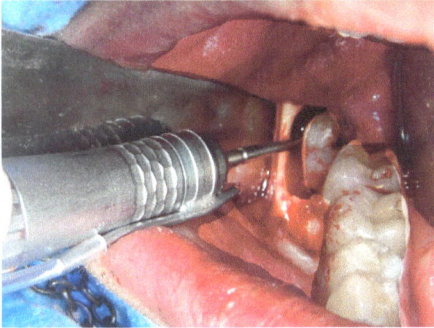

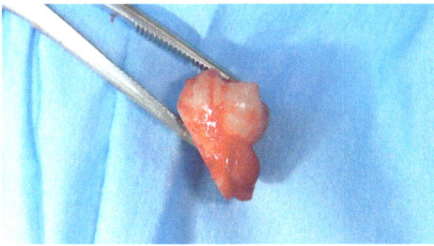

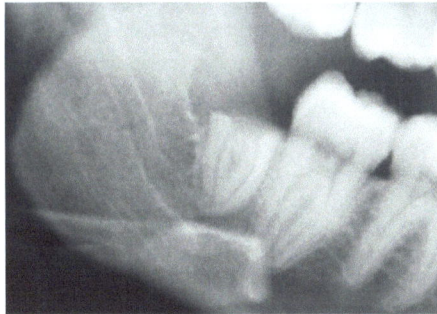

Coronectomy. The root is closely associated with the inferior dental bundle. A gutter of bone is removed buccally to gain access and the crown is removed, leaving most of the root with no risk to the nerve.

may become carious themselves. In any of these cases surgical removal is indicated. There is very little indication for removal of unerupted third molars; they rarely cause pathology unless associated with a cyst or are in the line of a mandibular fracture.

Each tooth that is listed for surgery should have the reason recorded in the patient's notes and decisions should be made according to the recommendations of NICE, the National Institute for Health and Care Excellence (Guidance on the extraction of wisdom teeth www.nice.org.uk). These are only guidelines so may be varied from in individual cases but the reason must be justifiable and recorded. During the consultation the patient should have the risks and benefits explained to them so that they may give informed consent for the procedure. Normally the patient should be listed for the surgical extractions to be carried out under local anaesthesia; sedation may be used for those who are apprehensive. Many surgeons carry out the surgery under general anaesthesia on a 'day-stay' basis; it is often used for bilateral extractions as there is only one recovery period for the patient.

When assessing the patient consideration should be given to the angulation of the tooth. Mesioangular (crown angled forward) are the easiest to remove, followed by deeper vertical teeth with distoangular (crown angled distally) impactions the most difficult. Obviously superficially placed teeth are easier to remove than deep. The 'difficulty' of removal relates to the amount of bone which will need removal and the ease of access.

We mentioned the NICE guidelines for removal of third molars. The National Institute for Health and Care Excellence (NICE) publication 'Technology Appraisal Guidance: on the Extraction of Wisdom Teeth'

It lays down sensible guidelines on when third molars should be removed and recommends no prophylactic surgery where there was no disease and no symptoms; it is a sensible disincentive to unnecessary surgery.

When first published in 2000 NICE very reasonably intended to review the guidance when the results of two expected controlled clinical trials were published. However these trials did not materialise so there was no review.

Recently it has been suggested that much of the third molar surgery stopped by NICE was needed eventually and was thus carried out on patients at an older age and that they suffered greater side effects and complications. Furthermore non removal of asymptomatic mesioangular impacted teeth predisposed to caries in the second molar which would not occur had the third molar been removed earlier. Clinical guidelines in other countries vary from that of NICE. In 2014 NICE reviewed the issues and decided not to vary its guidance but since then the

Faculty of Dental Surgery of the Royal College of Surgeons of England has published - Parameters of care for patients undergoing mandibular third molar surgery (www.rcseng.ac.uk).

It would not be necessary to have an intimate knowledge of the aforementioned lengthy document at undergraduate level. But where a patient has a part erupted mesioangular impacted third molar and poor oral hygiene with demineralisation of the distal of the second molar, then removal of the third molar should be discussed and possibly recommended to them.

Sometimes an upper tooth may be left unopposed after the removal of a lower or may be buccally placed or over-erupted. This may be sufficient justification for its removal and should produce minimal side effects and complications.

11 Ectopic Canines

Upper canine teeth are prone to become ectopic and are second only to third molars in the propensity to do so. The reasons for this are unclear but perhaps it is because they start their development far from their optimal final destination. Ectopic upper canines can cause resorption of the incisor teeth or produce an unacceptable appearance.

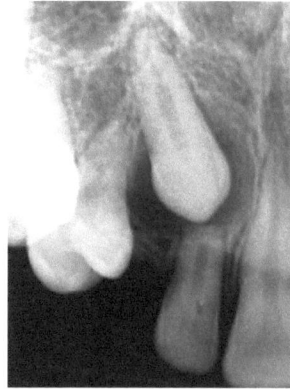

Resorption of a lateral incisor by an ectopic canine

The permanent upper canine teeth should normally become palpable in the upper buccal sulcus at the age of 10 or 11 years of age. Dentists should palpate for them in their child patients as a routine. They should suspect ectopic development if they are not palpable, if there is asymmetry between sides or the adjacent teeth are splayed apart. In these circumstances the child should be referred to an orthodontist for their opinion.

Ectopic canines are twice more likely to develop into a malposition on the palatal side of the dental arch than on the buccal side. The position of the unerupted tooth can be ascertained with X-rays using the horizontal parallax technique where an anterior occlusal and a periapical X-ray image are made and the position of canine relative to the other teeth can be visualised. The most accurate way of visualising the position is with a cone beam CT scan and

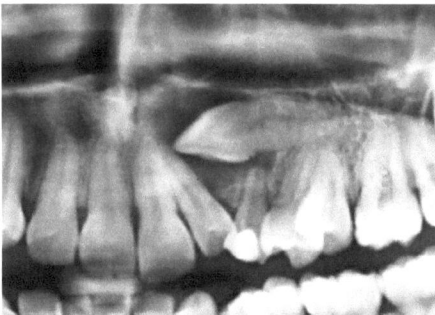

Detail from a panoral radiograph showing ectopic canine with follicular enlargement and displacement of adjacent teeth

this is used sometimes, particularly if root resorption of standing teeth is suspected, but in most cases it is not because the extra information provided is not warranted by the higher dose of radiation necessary.

If the canine is seen to be causing resorption of the permanent incisors then it should be removed to prevent further damage. It is rare for resorption to occur after the age of 14 so where patients present after this age they can be reassured with some degree of confidence.

Treatment for this problem is not essential. In some cases the distal of the lateral incisor will contact the mesial of the permanent first premolar giving a satisfactory appearance. Where canines are ectopic they should be reviewed radiographically to ensure there is not damage to the incisors up to the age of 15 after which this is most unlikely. Sometimes active treatment is not required because the patient is not concerned about the appearance or they have an otherwise poor dentition, and cannot maintain the oral hygiene standard or time commitment required for orthodontics. Sometimes the ectopic canine is in a position which is unamenable to orthodontic alignment, particularly if it is high above the apices of the adjacent teeth or close to the midline of the palate. Such an unerupted canine would only need removal if the follicle becomes cystic; otherwise it can remain in situ.

The first line of management will be to remove the deciduous canine tooth as in some cases this may encourage the permanent tooth to erupt into a normal position. However in many cases where an unacceptable aesthetic outcome is likely then orthodontics may be needed; in this case the orthodontist will request surgical help.

In some cases the tooth is uncovered surgically, a flap is raised and bone removed to expose the tooth and a temporary pack placed to discourage the soft tissue healing over it. This may encourage the tooth to erupt and it may then be guided into the optimal position in the dental arch with orthodontics. In many cases an orthodontic bracket will be attached to the tooth to pull it down; this may be done by the surgeon at the time of uncovering the tooth or later by the orthodontist when the tooth is visible. This is known as the 'open' technique.

The alternative 'closed' technique is where the surgeon uncovers the tooth and attaches an orthodontic bracket with a chain attached and then closes the wound. The orthodontist will then pull the tooth into position, having created sufficient space in the dental arch to move it to.

The surgery is normally carried out using general anaesthesia as a 'day case'. It normally involves raising a flap of palate which requires some controlled force. Bupivacaine and adrenaline local anaesthetic is normally infiltrated to give post-operative analgesia and decrease bleeding; lidocaine can be used but bupivacaine gives longer lasting analgesia. The position of the tooth to be uncovered can be ascertained beforehand using the parallax X-ray method as described above. However it is usually easily found clinically. Most teeth will be on the palatal side and will probably be visible as a bulge in the palate or be palpable. If it is not visible or palpable on either side the tooth might be felt through the mucosa palatally with a sharp probe or needle. If not, a palatal

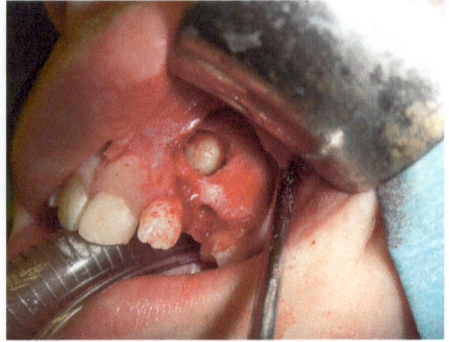

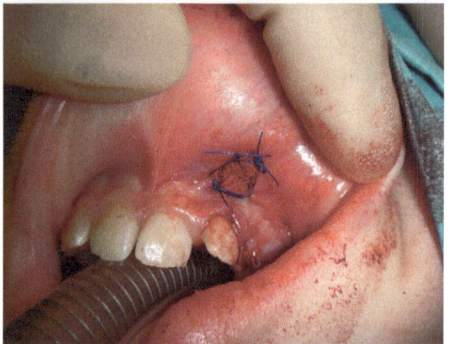

An ectopic canine has been exposed and the wound closed around a pack to uncover the tooth. The pack is removed a couple of weeks later and if necessary the orthodontist can attach a bracket. This is the 'open' technique

flap should be raised and in the possible situation where it is not found palatally, because it is in the line of the arch, a buccal flap may be also raised without detriment.

Teeth other than canines or third molars may sometimes remain unerupted. Generally these are usually not removed unless there is a specific reason to do so. Sometimes the follicle becomes enlarged leading to a dentigerous cyst, in which case tooth and cyst should be surgically removed. Sometimes unerupted teeth may weaken the jaw and present themselves when it is fractured, in which case it is usually removed at the time of surgery for the fracture.

Unerupted or supernumerary teeth may sometimes lead to interference with the normal eruption such as a mesiodens between the incisor teeth; removal is usually requested by an orthodontist.

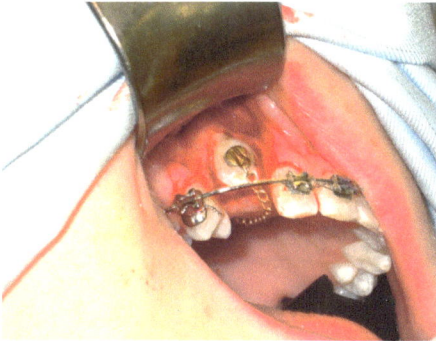

The 'closed' technique. The tooth has been uncovered and a bracket and a chain attached. The flap will be closed and the orthodontist can now pull the tooth into place.

Examination tip:

▪ Know the normal age of eruption of the permanent teeth and be prepared to answer questions about dental development (particularly of the canines) when presented with panoral images

▪ Be aware of the indications for canine uncovering or removal

▪ Know that canines should be palpated for at age 10 or 11 and referred to an orthodontist if necessary

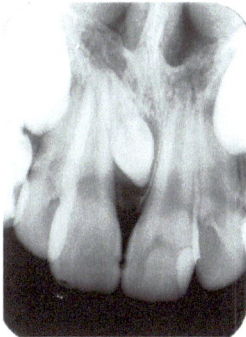

Left: a mesiodens. This can be left alone if it does not interfere with the incisor eruption

Below: a different mesiodens at operation. It is interfering with the incisor eruption.

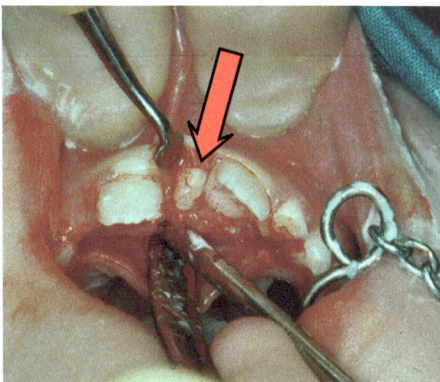

12 Post-operative Advice and Analgesia

Following surgery the patient should be given an absorbent sterile surgical swab to bite on until the bleeding has stopped, usually about 10 minutes. After that they should be seated comfortably and kept for a while longer to ensure they are comfortable and bleeding has not re-started.

Post-operative instructions should be given verbally and in writing. The patient should be warned about the possibility of swelling or bruising (which may be caused by bleeding into the soft tissue) and that their saliva is likely to be stained with blood for up to two days.

They should be given some surgical swabs to bite on for 20 minutes should there be any recurrence of bleeding and details of how they may get assistance from you should any bleeding occur which they cannot control in this manner. This should include an emergency telephone number.

The patient should avoid rinsing the mouth for 24 hours but after that they can gently rinse the area with warm salty mouthwashes 3 times daily for 3 days. Oral hygiene measures should avoid traumatising the operation site and hygiene may be aided with gentle chlorhexidine mouth washes. They should be advised that some limitation of mouth opening may occur and that they should chew on the opposite side.

Post-operative soreness or pain are unavoidable. The emotional component of pain and the response to surgery may be tempered with accurate information about what the patient may experience during and afterwards; this has been shown to help reduce pain.

Patients should be recommended to take analgesics regularly for two days after minor oral surgery and advised that post-operative pain is always better managed when anticipated by taking medication regularly, rather than reacted to by taking medication in response to pain. The first dose should be taken before the local anaesthetic has worn off.

Non-steroidal anti-inflammatory drugs will help by reducing inflammation as well as modulating the pain perception pathways and Ibuprofen taken as 400 mg. taken every 4 to 6 hours with a maximum of 2400 mg. in 24 hours is effective after

Medications used for pain after minor oral surgery

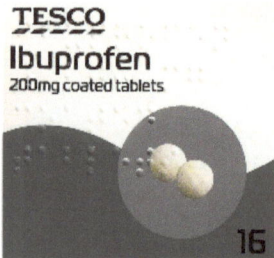

Our recommended first choice. Available from the shelf from supermarkets and most grocery stores. These were £0.40p for 16 tablets.

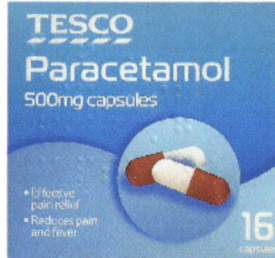

The most commonly used and our recommended choice where NSAID are contra-indicated. These were £0.39p for 16 tablets

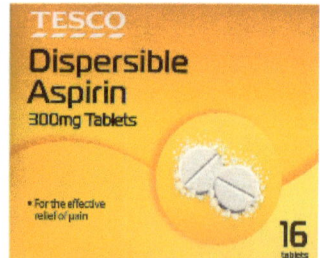

Common and dependable. £0.55p for 16 tablets from the supermarket

minor oral surgery. Paracetamol is probably slightly less effective but is the most commonly used drug. It is not a NSAID and can be particularly useful where they are contraindicated. 1000 mg. Taken 4 to 6 hourly with a maximum of 4000 mg. in 24 hours.

There is good evidence that Ibuprofen 200 mg. and Paracetamol 500 mg. taken in combination 3 times a day are the most effective. Aspirin may also be used, best in dispersible form, 600 mg. 4 hourly, maximum 4000 mg. daily.

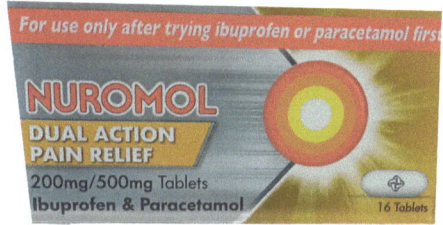

Studies have shown Ibuprofen and Paracetmol combined is most effective for pain after minor oral surgery. We would suggest this for patients who report unacceptable pain with monotherapy. This packet was £5 for 16 tablets.

Post-operative instructions following surgical procedures in the mouth

In the next 24 hours:

- Do not rinse your mouth out for the rest of the day or spit.
- Clean your teeth but do not interfere with the surgical area.
- Take it easy for the rest of the day; no physical activity.
- Be careful not to bite your lip or tongue.
- Do not be alarmed if you can feel sharp fragments around the socket; they will disappear.

Rinsing:

- After 24 hours take warm salt mouth baths, (one teaspoon of salt to a glass of warm water) every 2 - 4 hours for the next 7 days especially after food and at bed times.

Bleeding:

- Nothing to eat or drink until the numbness has worn off.
- Nothing too hot or cold for the rest of the day (as this may start the bleeding off).

- A soft diet is advisable for the first few days.

Pain relief:

- Pain and swelling is normal after an operation.
- For pain relief you are advised to take appropriate pain killers (as advised by your dentist/pharmacist).
- Take all antibiotics as prescribed.
- Do not drink alcohol with antibiotic Metronidazole (Flagyl).

Sutures:

- These dissolve and last 1-2 weeks

Other problems:

- Many people suffer sensitivity of the teeth next to the sockets. Clean well and the problem will resolve itself with time.
- No smoking for 48 hours after the procedure.

Medications used for pain after minor oral surgery

Medication	Use	Contra-indications	Side effects
Ibuprofen 400 mg. 4 hrly max 2400 mg. in 24 hrs	Most effective first line drug. Is a NSAID	Allergy to NSAID History gastric ulceration Renal impairment Uncontrolled asthma Bleeding disorders Anti-coagulants	Many but unlikely with just two days of treatment. Chiefly gastro intestinal upsets
Paracetamol 1000 mg. 4-6 hrly max 4000 mg. in 24 hr	Not a NSAID Not quite as effective as Ibuprofen but more commonly used. Very dangerous in overdose	High alcohol intake Liver disease Must not take more than max dose - high risk of fatal liver failure	Well tolerated Advise no more than 3 alcoholic drinks per day
Ibuprofen/Paracetamol combination 200/500 x 3 daily	Cochrane review has reported this regime to be the most effective	As above	As above
Aspirin 600 mg. 4 hrly max 4000 mg. in 24 hr	Is a NSAID Dispersible form reported most effective	Allergy to NSAID History gastric bleeding Bleeding disorders Anti-coagulents Asthma related to previous NSAID Avoid in late pregnancy Not for children - Reye's syndrome	Gastro intestinal upsets Gastric bleeding but probably only with chronic use

13 Complications

A complication is an adverse event which may increase the morbidity of a patient following any treatment, most commonly, but not necessarily, a surgical operation. As surgeons we seek to minimise the risk of complications by good pre-operative planning, sound surgery and meticulous post-operative care and cross infection control.

Bleeding

Bleeding is a normal side effect of oral surgery and the patient should have an explanation that bleeding into the mouth will always occur afterwards. Unlike soft tissue surgery carried out through a skin incision there will always be bone exposed when teeth are removed and this will bleed into the void left by an extraction. Blood will escape through the socket and into the mouth either directly or through the mucosa margins if a soft tissue flap has been raised. It is desirable that any blood does escape into the mouth as any accumulation beneath the periosteum will cause swelling and bruising.

However bleeding becomes a complication if the patient returns after the event or if bleeding is difficult to control at the time of the surgery. Bleeding that occurs within a couple of days of surgery is called 'reactionary haemorrhage'. If it occurs later, it may be initiated by infection and is termed 'secondary haemorrhage' although this is unusual in oral surgery. Frequently the patient will be alarmed or distressed and the situation often looks much worse than it is as a small amount of blood appears significant when mixed with saliva which has been stimulated by the operation and by frequent spitting. Below we have listed the procedures you should follow for a patient who presents with reactionary bleeding after dental extraction or other minor oral surgery. We will assume it is for a patient you have not previously known so as to include everything that might be expected

---

Complications of minor oral surgery

Bleeding

- Immediate or delayed
- Swelling and bruising (side effects)

Infection

- Post extraction osteitis (dry socket)
- Spreading infection

Antral

- Oro-antral communication
- Tooth displaced into antrum

Nerve Damage

- Lingual
- Inferior dental

Bone Necrosis

- Medication induced
- Osteoradionecrosis

Iatrogenic

- Damage to adjacent teeth or restorations
- Jaw fracture

---

of you in an examination.

Note that bleeding in patients taking anticoagulants or anti-platelet medication can almost always be managed with these local measures without altering their medication, if their dosage is correct. In practice non-steroidal anti-inflammatories rarely cause any significant problem in oral surgery (but you should always mention them in examinations).

Swelling and bruising

These can also be considered as side effects if small. Swelling can be caused by the acute trauma of tissue manipulation if the surgery has been difficult and prolonged and some patients are more susceptible than others. Bruising is caused by the breakdown products of haemoglobin and can be caused by bleeding into the soft

Procedure for post-op bleeding

1. Seat the patient comfortably, slightly reclined in a dental chair with a good light and efficient suction.

2. Remove anything loose from the mouth such as swabs, tissue paper, dentures, and suck out any clots and identify the source of bleeding. Place a rolled up swab over the wound and get the patient to bite on it firmly for 20 minutes.

3. As best as possible take a history from the patient with help from any accompanying person. In particular: a history of the extraction/surgery, when, where, difficulty, post-op instructions.

4. Take a medical history in particular of previous surgery/bleeding problem, history of bruising, family history of bleeding, drug history particularly of anticoagulant, antiplatelet medication and non-steroidal anti-inflammatories.

4. Assess the patient's general condition. Are they anxious/distressed, pale or have tachycardia? These may occur after significant blood loss, although this is very rare from minor oral surgery; blood pressure is a poor indicator of blood loss as physiological compensation occurs producing a normal pressure even after significant loss. Anxiety may cause tachycardia and hypertension making bleeding worse.

5. After 20 minutes remove swabs and reassess; this might have been enough and you can discharge the patient with a supply of swabs and instructions.

6. Otherwise apply pressure across the wound with gloved fingers; if this stops the bleeding it is probably oozing from soft tissues and suturing may help; topically applied tranexamic acid can also be used. Bleeding from bone is best dealt with by packing with oxidised cellulose gauze. In practice we prefer to pack and suture, keep the patient biting for another 20 minutes and then keep them for observation for another half hour before discharging.

7. Heavy or uncontrolled bleeding should be referred to hospital.

8. Patients with inappropriate bleeding should be requested to see their GP for coagulation screening. Patients taking warfarin should have their INR checked to ensure it is not outside the therapeutic range (chapter 02).

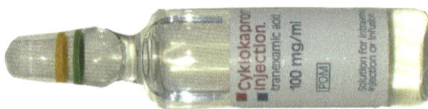

Tranexamic acid is used in hospitals, can be applied topically on a swab to reduce bleeding. It works by inhibiting fibrinolysis. It can be given intravenously but should be used with care in the elderly as it can predispose to stroke.

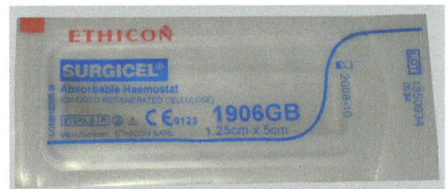

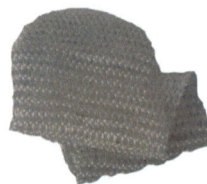

Oxidised cellulose gauze is packed tightly into a wound to stop bleeding from the bone. It will later resorb.

tissues. It is unusual in minor oral surgery as the bleeding normally occurs into the mouth. Occasionally bleeding may be severe into the soft tissues and form as a haematoma which is a collection of blood. This is very unusual after minor oral surgery but will result in swelling and bruising. The bruising normally moves down the neck under the influence of gravity.

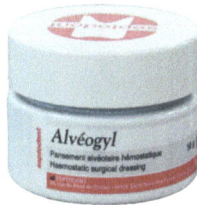

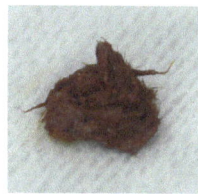

Alvogyl contains Eugenol (analgesic), Butamben, (local anaesthetic) and Iodoform (anti-microbial).

Infection

All oral surgery wounds will be 'contaminated' by the normal oral flora but in most cases there will be no untoward effects because the patient's immune systems are able to deal with it. A contamination becomes an 'infection' when the organisms get the upper hand causing unwanted signs and symptoms such as prolonged pain, swelling or suppuration with pus.

In most cases the clinical scenario will be a post-operative osteitis also known as 'dry socket'. This is more common in the mandible, in smokers and where oral hygiene is poor. The patient will present with pain becoming worse rather than better a few days after the surgery. Examination reveals no organising blood clot in the wound but rather it is 'dry' with visible exposed bone.

Most cases are self-limiting but because of the severe pain are usually treated by irrigating debris out of the bony socket with warm saline and packing with Alvogyl®, a proprietary preparation containing an analgesic, a local anaesthetic, and an anti-microbial. Sometimes a second dressing may be needed and recalcitrant cases may be helped by curetting the infected cancellous bone at the margin of the socket under local anaesthesia to make it bleed and help form a clot. Antibiotics are inappropriate as there is no spreading infection and systemic upset. Most post-operative osteitis occurs in the mandible.

Occasionally post-operative infection may lead to spreading infection which may form a collection of pus in the submandibular area beneath the mylohyoid muscle. This is rare and usually occurs after surgical removal of third molars, an area from where pus can get beneath the mylohyoid. Here hospital admission and intravenous antibiotics may be appropriate followed by draining of the pus.

Oro-antral communication

The upper second premolars and molars may be close to the maxillary antrum but the first and second molars usually have roots that are intimately associated or protruding into the antrum. Removal of these teeth may therefore result in a communication which in the worst case can lead to fluid coming out of the nose when drinking and sinusitis with pain.

Patients should be warned of the possibility when these teeth are to be removed. After the surgery they should be advised to avoid blowing their nose or sneezing (if possible) which will raise the pressure in the antrum and disturb the clot. However in most cases, even where there is a communication, the socket will fill with a blood clot and normal healing and bone formation will occur, producing no untoward effect.

However in a small minority of cases a communication will persist into a fistula (an epithelial lined tract between two epithelial lined cavities) with the above mentioned consequences. In this case the patient will need surgery to remove the epithelial tract, close the soft tissue over the communication and clean out the antrum. The latter can now be done by an ENT surgeon with an endoscopy; a scope is used to make an antrostomy thorough the lateral wall of the nasal cavity below the anatomical ostium (to encourage drainage) and wash out the sinus.

Occasionally a root of an upper molar may be displaced into the antrum during an injudicious attempt to remove a root that has broken off during an extraction. This may well lead to a communication as healing will be compromised by infection, but it will almost certainly lead to a florid sinusitis with pain and discharge into the mouth through the wound. The root should be retrieved. Initially this should be attempted with a high volume suction tip. It may also be done surgically through the mouth by extending the surgical wound, but this risks making a larger communication with the antrum. The root may be retrieved via a Caldwell-Luc approach from higher up in the maxilla through the thin bone at the canine fossa above and slightly behind the upper canine. We would do this as an 'urgent' procedure i.e. within a couple of days before the antrum fills up with polyps and infection which would produce a sinusitis, and lead to a discharging communication into the mouth developing and require an antrostomy to encourage nasal drainage of the antrum rather than into the mouth. If a displaced root is small an ENT surgeon may be able to remove it with an endoscope.

Nerve Damage

In theory it is possible to damage the mental nerve when operating on the lower premolars as it emerges from the mental foramen close to the apices of these teeth. You should mention the sensory disturbance that may result when asked in examinations but in practice the operator will have to be pretty clumsy to cause this.

The greatest risk of nerve injury is to the lingual nerve during removal of lower third molars leading to sensory deficit in the tongue. Most cases are temporary and

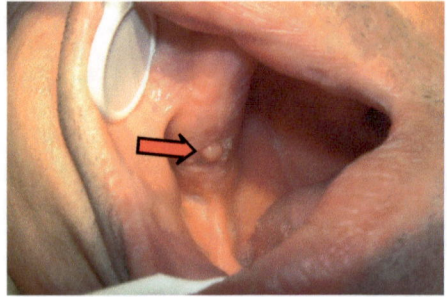

A persistent oro-antral communication on the alveolus after upper 6 was removed. The patient could blow air through the hole and he had sinusitis. It was closed surgically and an antrostomy carried out to allow the sinus to drain.

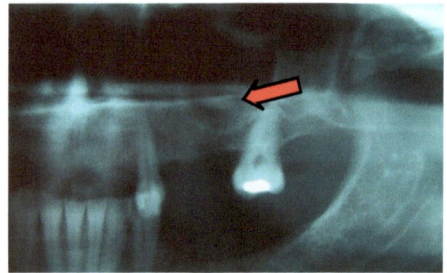

Part of an panoral radiograph showing a displaced palatal root from upper first molar

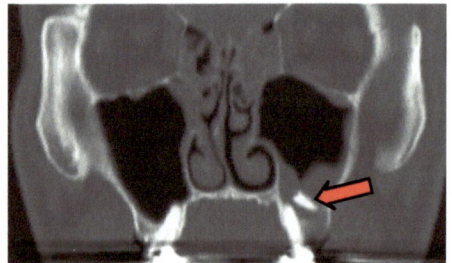

A coronal CT scan shows the root and a profuse inflammatory proliferation of the antral lining as sinusitis develops. Note the proximity of the palatal root of the 6 to the antrum on the other side.

caused by stretching the nerve if a lingual retractor is used. However it is possible to cause permanent damage with a surgical bur and this can be a significant disability to the patient. The root of lower third molars can be very close to the inferior dental nerve in

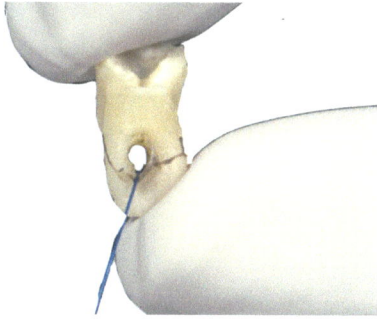

The roots of this third molar surrounded the inferior dental canal. Very unusual.

the mandibular canal and this can be injured during their removal (chapter 10). Should this occur it is likely to cause only temporary sensory disturbance and if permanent is less likely to be a disability. Cone beam CT scanning may be used to demonstrate the relationship of the roots to the ID bundle and the morphology of the roots; it uses only a low dose of radiation. However it's use has not shown to have had any beneficial effect on damage to the inferior dental nerve to justify the expense and radiation received; (see: Journal of Craniomaxillofacial Surgery 2015; 43: 2158-2167. Also: Parameters of care for patients undergoing mandibular third molar surgery. Royal College of Surgeons. 2020 (www.rcs.ac.uk).

Bone Necrosis

The potential for bone necrosis should be anticipated before treatment is started with either medication or radiotherapy that can cause it (chapter 02). However there will be some patients where extractions are unavoidable after therapy has been carried out. In most cases this will be in patients who have received oral bisphosphonates for osteopenia or osteoporosis or other antiresorptives for osteoporosis which may have been given intravenously.

The medication in this form is considered low risk and the incidence will be low but the prevalence will be high due to the large numbers of post-menopausal women taking medication for many years.

It is important not to confuse the clinical appearance of bone necrosis with a normal post extraction osteitis (dry socket) and curette the socket to induce healing as this will make it worse. Patients should be referred to an oral and maxillofacial surgeon or oral surgeon as they will see a large number of these patients. Management is normally expectant. Debridement and removal of exfoliating dead bone may be appropriate, but surgery is often unhelpful. Patients can usually can expect to discharge pus permanently with antibiotics reserved for where there is severe spreading cellulitis.

Osteoradionecrosis is a miserable affliction leading to infection, pain,

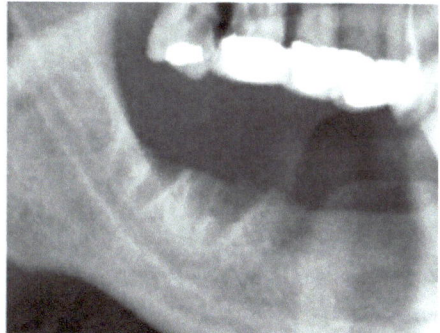

Patient presented with submandibular swelling and discomfort from where lower molars had been removed over a year previously. The X-ray showed the extraction sockets.

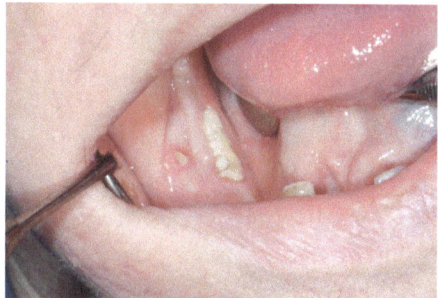

There was necrotic bone erupting through the mucosa. She had been having bisphosphonate infusions for metastatic breast cancer.

pathological fracture and salivary fistulae to the skin. Patients will have been assessed by a cancer team pre-treatment and an oral and maxillofacial surgeon or a restorative dentist will have prescribed removal of teeth associated with the radiotherapy. More conservative regimes where teeth are preserved can end in disaster. Patients with osteoradionecrosis should be seen by their cancer management team. Surgery will involve vascularised bone grafts.

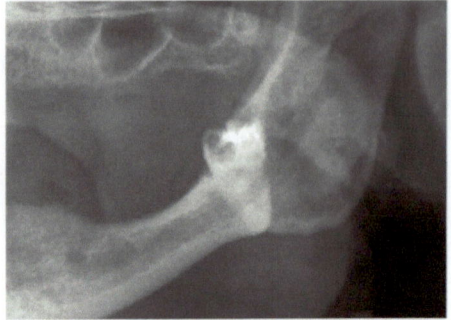

Part of a panoral radiograph showing a previously unerupted third molar which is now breeching the mucosa and causing discomfort below a lower denture. The mandible is significantly resorbed and removal carries a high risk of fracture.

Damage to adjacent teeth or restorations

This is most likely to occur if the restorations are already defective, the adjacent tooth is already loose or damaged, or the operator is careless. But should always mention in examinations. However it will be difficult to elevate a mesioangular impacted lower third molar without damaging an overhanging restoration in the distal of the adjacent lower molar. In this case the patient should be warned the restoration is over-hanging and will need replacing afterwards.

Fracture

It is possible to fracture a mandible during minor oral surgery but in all the cases we have seen there has been some degree of poor planning or carelessness.

14 Local Anaesthesia

The vast majority of oral surgery is carried out by using local anaesthetic. We will discuss the background information necessary for examinations but not repeat the injection techniques which are best taught by practical instruction.

Lidnocaine with adrenaline
(often called lignocaine)

The mainstay of local anaesthesia for oral surgery is lidocaine 2% with the vasoconstrictor adrenaline at a concentration of 1:80000. Like all the local anaesthetic agents we use it is an amide; it is highly effective and gives good pulpal anaesthesia for about an hour and soft tissue for about two hours if given as an infiltration and slightly longer for an inferior dental nerve block.

Local anaesthetics are vasodilators and they would soon diffuse away were it not for the vasoconstrictor which prolongs the action to the aforementioned times and also helps to reduce bleeding which is an added advantage for surgery.

Injected adrenaline will have an effect directly on the heart causing tachycardia, increased cardiac output and possibly palpations so, for nerve blocks at least, we inject slowly with an aspirating syringe to reduce the risk of intravascular injection.

As an approximate 'rule of thumb' we would give up to a maximum of 7 x 2.2 ml, cartridges if given slowly with an aspirating syringe. However if working on only one quadrant of the mouth you should never need more than four. Lidocaine is metabolised in the liver so this should be reduced in patients with severe liver disease. They will still need to have the same dose to make them numb but this should be limited to work on one quadrant of the mouth.

Prilocaine with felypressin

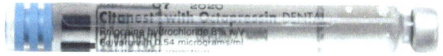

Prilocaine 3% with 0.54 micrograms/ml felypressin is sometimes used for patients with cardiac disease such as unstable angina (nowadays rare), uncontrolled hypertension (rare), recent acute cardiac events (such as myocardial infarction) and more commonly for patients who say for some reason they don't want adrenaline.

We believe that this is a less effective agent and gives a shorter anaesthetic time for both pulp and soft tissue. Patients who have had heart transplants will have a denervated heart and this will be very susceptible to adrenaline injection and this may be a good reason to use prilocaine with felypressin. It has been alleged that felypressin may induce labour.

Articaine with adrenaline

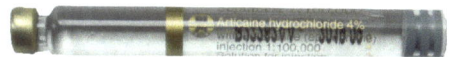

Articaine 4% with 1:100,000 adrenaline is used by some who believe it is a more effective agent than lidocaine with adrenaline. If so this may be related to its higher concentration. It may be used in children's dentistry to infiltrate for mandibular molars to avoid an inferior dental nerve block. It does have a longer duration of action for pulpal and soft tissue anaesthesia. It tends not to be used for inferior dental nerve blocks because of the long soft tissue anaesthesia and because it has been alleged to have a higher incidence of nerve damage. We do not believe that buccal infiltration of articaine to avoid inferior dental nerve blocks is adequate for oral surgery on mandibular molar teeth. Teeth with inflamed pulps and/or acutely infected are more difficult to anaesthetise. We describe how we deal with this situation with lidocaine and adrenaline in chapter 17.

Bupivacaine with adrenaline

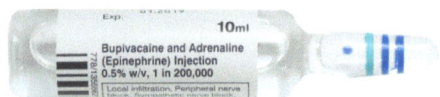

Bupivacaine 0.5% with 1:200,000 adrenaline is a long acting anaesthetic which we infiltrate around the operation site for patients receiving both minor and major oral surgery under general anaesthetic. It may give soft tissue anaesthesia for up to 6 hours. The local anaesthetic will allow the anaesthetist to give the patient a lighter anaesthetic than otherwise, the adrenaline will decrease bleeding and the patient will have no post-operative pain for several hours.

Some patients complain that they have an allergy to local anaesthetic or adrenaline. These are rarely true 'allergies' i.e. immunological in aetiology. Most are autonomic reactions such as syncope, tachycardia or sweating. Occasionally a reaction may be due to overdose or as a result of inadvertent intravascular injection. Patients should be referred to an allergy clinic to ascertain whether there is a true allergy.

Complications of Local Anaesthesia

- **Syncope** (simple faint): caused by anxiety + pain/discomfort on injection

- **Other psychological reactions**: hyperventilation, nausea, tachycardia, palpations

- **Toxic effects:** from severe overdose or intravascular injection. Includes lightheadedness, slurred speech, disorientation, muscle twitching (very rare)

- **Persistent paraesthesia**: from hitting the nerve during ID block (almost always recovers) is associated with articaine and prilocaine

- **Trismus**: from a haematoma in the medial pterygoid muscle caused during ID block

- **True allergy:** urticaria, swelling bronchospasm (very rare)

Examination tips:

- Know how to manage a faint if it occurs during administration of local anaesthesia

- Know how to manage a patient who alleges an allergy to local anaesthesia

- Be able to demonstrate how to assemble a local anaesthetic syringe for use

- Learn the techniques for local anaesthetic administration (not covered in this book).

15 Conscious Sedation

Sedation is defined as: -

'a technique in which the use of a drug or drugs produces a state of depression of the central nervous system enabling treatment to be carried out, but during which verbal contact with the patient is maintained throughout the period of sedation.

For dental sedation the drugs and techniques used should carry a margin of safety wide enough to render loss of consciousness unlikely.'

(Quoted from: Standards for Conscious Sedation in the Provision of Dental Care - Dental faculties of the Royal Colleges of Surgeons and the Royal College of Anaesthetists)

Sedation is particularly appropriate in dentistry for the management of patients who may be phobic, have a pronounced gag reflex or who require a lengthy procedure. For the majority of routine restorative work it is in the patient's best interest to use alternative behaviour strategies to encourage them to accept their routine care using local anaesthesia alone.

However most oral surgery procedures are likely to be a solitary experience for the patient as well as being more prolonged and uncomfortable than their routine dental treatment. Sedation will make it more acceptable and less unpleasant. In many cases a nervous patient may request a general anaesthetic and sedation will be an acceptable alternative which is readily available in a primary care setting and will be less expensive to provide.

As an undergraduate you will be expected to know about the two techniques of sedation which are most frequently used in dental care: inhalation sedation using nitrous oxide and oxygen, which is most commonly used for children and restorative treatment, and intravenous sedation using the benzodiazepine midazolam, most

---

Conscious Sedation Indications

• Facilitates dental treatment for a patient who might otherwise be incapable due to phobia or pronounced gag reflex

• Makes the procedure less unpleasant, particularly for longer procedures

• Causes amnesia

• Is more cost-effective than general anaesthesia because:

  ▪it may be given by operator

  ▪it can be used in primary care setting

Conscious Sedation Risks

• Over sedation could lead to hypoxia → myocardial excitability or depression → cardiac event

• Over sedation could lead to compromised gag reflex → inhalation of saliva, blood, tooth fragment or materials → bronchopneumonia or lung abscess

• Patients might come to physical harm if they drive a vehicle or carry out any activity requiring judgement in the period after treatment before sedation has completely worn off

• Some patients can experience sexual hallucinations with midazolam

---

commonly used for adults undergoing oral surgery.

The so called 'alternative techniques' are reserved for use by dentists with specific post-graduate training or, more usually, anaesthetists who often use a combination of drugs, particularly midazolam and propofol which does have certain particular advantages.

Dentists may give inhalation sedation with nitrous oxide/oxygen or intravenous with midazolam as well as operating, provided they are assisted by a nurse trained to monitor the patient and another to assist them with the procedure.

Sedation produces depression of the central nervous system but this must be limited to the extent that the patient is able to retain their vital reflexes including swallowing and be able to communicate with the sedationist throughout the procedure. This should leave a wide margin of safety between a sedated patient who will accept treatment and an unconscious one. This ideal can be routinely accomplished with inhaled nitrous oxide/oxygen or intravenous midazolam.

Inhalation Sedation

Nitrous oxide is an effective depressant of the central nervous system as well as having analgesic properties. When inhaled it acts quickly and the depression is reversed quickly when it is withdrawn. It appears to have no toxic side effects and after treatment the patient's cognitive ability quickly returns to normal and they can resume their usual activities.

The inhalation sedation technique starts with the patient being given 100% oxygen through a mask over their nose for a couple of minutes and then nitrous oxide is introduced at 10% for a minute and then 20,

25 and 30% at minute intervals as the level of sedation is monitored by observation of the patient's response.

As the patient becomes more sedated they will become more relaxed, the rate at which they blink their eyes will decrease, they will assume a glazed appearance, their responses will be reduced and they will appear flushed and warm. Their speech will become slurred and their eyes will show ptosis (drooping of the upper eyelids). The operator should talk to the patient throughout to help relax and reassure them but also to judge their response to the nitrous oxide and judge at what stage treatment can start. They should retain their normal reflexes including swallowing.

When the treatment has finished the patient is given 100% oxygen for two minutes, after which they should have returned to normal function. In successive treatment sessions the patient may be given a lower concentration of nitrous oxide as they become more confident and possibly weaned off sedation entirely.

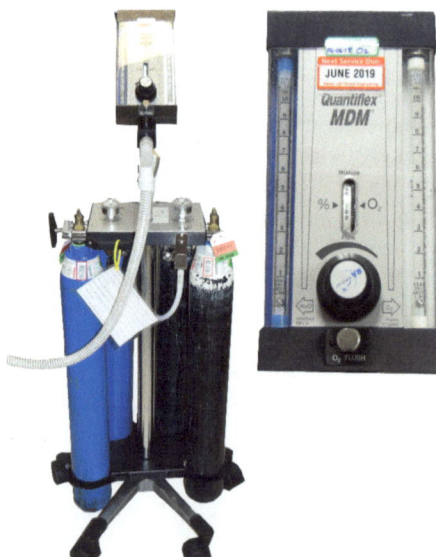

Left: inhalation sedation machine. The gas goes to a nasal cannula in the patient via the tube on the left. Right: detail of the control for adjusting and monitoring the nitrous oxide/oxygen mixture.

Intravenous sedation

Midazolam is a water soluble benzodiazepine which is given intravenously and is the most frequently used agent for sedation in oral surgery. It is sedative, anxiolytic, causes a profound amnesia and has a short half-life making it ideal for oral surgery sedation. Its effect can be quickly reversed with flumazenil but this is not routinely needed because midazolam has a short half-life so patients recover quickly without it. Flumazenil is kept available for an accidental overdose situation, which should never occur as midazolam is administered carefully and slowly in increments.

Midazolam has no analgesic properties so patients sometimes flinch a little when the local anaesthetic injection is administered and it has been known to produce sexual hallucinations so the operator/sedationist should never be left alone with the patient before, during or after the treatment. There should always be two nurses present anyway, one to monitor the patient and another to assist with the surgery.

Midazolam is given through an intravenous cannula, most usually inserted into a suitable vein in the back of the hand and adequately secured. A trained nurse should monitor the patient by recording their level of consciousness, respiratory rate and oxygen saturation using a pulse oximeter from which a baseline reading has been taken at the start. Oxygen and flumazenil should be available to use if the patient should become over sedated, although this is unlikely; midazolam has a high therapeutic window.

Once the patient is adequately prepared 2 mg are given slowly over 30 seconds followed by a 2 minute pause while the level of sedation is assessed clinically by the operator monitoring the signs, as above. The dose is then titrated upwards at the rate of 0.5 mgms. every 30 seconds until the desired level of sedation is reached. There

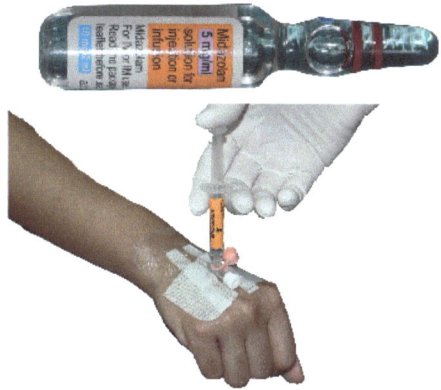

Midazolam is slowly titrated into an intravenous cannula sited in the back of the hand while the patient's response is observed

is a wide variation in the dose needed between individuals. Most patients will need between 2 and 7.5 mgms. The elderly should be given the initial and incremental doses more slowly.

In the unlikely event that the patient's oxygen saturation should fall or their respiration become too depressed the procedure should stop and they should be encouraged to breathe and given some oxygen through a nasal mask. Ultimately flumazenil could be given to reverse the sedation but you should be aware that flumazenil has a very short half life and a patient may sedate again after it has worn off.

After the procedure the patient should be recovered with a nurse and should go home accompanied by an adult who should receive all the post-operative advice and instructions verbally as well as in writing; the patient will still be amnesic. Most important is that they should not drive a vehicle or carry out any other potentially unsafe task for 48 hours.

Intravenous sedation can be less predictable in children and therefore it is generally not used. For children requiring dental extractions or other oral surgery it is most appropriate for an anaesthetist to

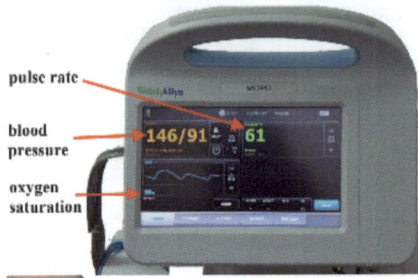

pulse rate

blood pressure

oxygen saturation

The pulse oximeter is attached to the pulp of a finger and together with a blood pressure cuff the machine will show blood pressure, pulse rate and oxygen saturation. The respiratory rate and depth of sedation is assessed by observation.

assess them; in most cases a general anaesthetic will be more appropriate.

Alternative Techniques

The so called 'alternative techniques' are not normally used by dental surgeons but can be with special training. They include oral sedation with the benzodiazepines temazepam or midazolam which may even be given intra nasally. However, mostly due to variation in individual response, these methods of administration are less predictable and therefore infrequently used.

Another alternative technique is the combination of the use of midazolam with the opiate fentanyl or the anaesthetic agent propofol. These techniques are unsuitable for use by an operator/sedationist in the dental surgery as it is less easy to titrate the doses and there will be a lower margin between moderate sedation and the patient becoming unconscious; they are usually used by anaesthetists in the operating theatre. The advantage is that the patient will be less responsive to pain and will not flinch when the local anaesthetic is administered and, where propofol is combined with midazolam, recovery from the sedation will be very rapid as the

midazolam may be given in very low doses; recovery from propofol is fast.

The most frequent reason we would ask an anaesthetist to give the sedation will be if the patient is not medically fit. The American Society of Anaesthetists in 1962 devised the Physical Status Classification System range from a Grade 1 (fit and healthy) to Grade 6 (dead). For a dentist to sedate a patient and act as operator the patient must fit ASA Grade 1 or 2 (see table). For patients with severe respiratory or cardiovascular disease or sleep apnoea an anaesthetist may sedate with propofol and midazolam, give oxygen via nasal cannulae and monitor them with ECG as well as pulse oximetry.

Assessment and Consent

The patient should be seen for an appointment before the surgery for assessment. At this stage the dentist should discuss and record the reasons for sedating the patient and any alternatives which might be acceptable to them. The assessment should include a full medical and dental history. Base line vital signs should be recorded including blood pressure, pulse and respiratory rates and oxygen saturation. The patient's ASA grading should be recorded. They should be given verbal and written instructions which should include the advice not to have alcohol or recreational drugs for 24 hours beforehand, to take their normal medication at the usual times and to be accompanied by a responsible adult who will escort them home, preferably by private car or taxi.

Consent for treatment should preferably be obtained on a day prior to the actual treatment when the patient is assessed for their oral and general medical state. This should be confirmed on the day of treatment. The patient should be given written information about sedation. If the patient is in pain and immediate treatment needed this ideal will not be possible. Adult patients receiving the usual moderate sedation for treatment will maintain their normal reflexes and swallowing ability so should not need to starve beforehand.

Whilst it is permissible for the operator to give the sedation they should have received training to do so and be accompanied by two nurses who have also received training. Dental nurses can take the National Examining Board for Dental Nurses certificate in Dental Sedation Nursing. One nurse should assist in the surgery and one should monitor the patient's vital signs and record them every 5 minutes. There should be appropriate recovery facilities. Afterwards the patient should remain at least an hour after the last dose of midazolam and until they can walk unaided and talk coherently. They should be accompanied home by a responsible adult.

Examination tip:

▪ Anticipate being asked to take a history and counsel a 'patient' (actor) presenting with severe anxiety over having a dental extraction and be able to discuss the techniques available to them.

16 General Anaesthesia

By the year 2000 there were concerns about the provision of general anaesthesia in primary dental care as there had been several deaths reported and many anaesthetics provided where there was no justifiable clinical need. The Department of Health publication of 'A conscious decision, a review of the use of general anaesthesia and conscious sedation in primary dental care' was published and since that time all general anaesthetics for dentistry must be provided in a hospital environment.

However there is still a high patient-driven demand for general anaesthesia for oral surgery in spite of the fact that it is less readily available. Individual decisions on whether an anaesthetic is provided will depend upon what facilities are available, patient anxiety, waiting times and, for children needing dental extractions, the number of teeth to be removed. Most single tooth extractions are driven by patient demand and anxiety rather than need.

However there is very little clinical need for general anaesthesia for oral surgery. Most treatment can be provided with local anaesthesia alone or supplemented with sedation for very anxious patients. The exceptions will be for those who are unable to cooperate, most of whom will be children needing multiple dental extractions or exposure of unerupted teeth as part of an orthodontic treatment plan. Intravenous drug abusers can be difficult to sedate reliably and this would be another good reason for a general anaesthetic to be provided rather than sedation. A lower threshold for providing an anaesthetic may be appropriate where the surgery is likely to be prolonged. Many adults will receive general anaesthetics for removal of impacted third molars, particularly if these are bilateral. However if the appropriate NICE guidelines are followed the need for bilateral surgery

General anaesthetic pre-operative checklist:
Record in the patient's notes:
• Treatment prescribed
• Why a general anaesthetic
• Alternatives have been discussed
• Full medical history
• Previous dental history
• Consent for treatment
• Patient accompanied with adult to look after them post op
• Told fluid, food & medication policy and why
• Given pre-op advice in writing to supplement oral instructions

should be infrequent and even then sedation may be used.

Before a patient is referred for surgery under general anaesthetic a full medical and dental history should be taken, including details of previous dental treatment and how that was delivered. The treatment needed should be clearly recorded; it should be discussed with the patient and consent obtained and consent form signed. There should be a record of why a general anaesthetic is being requested and what possible alternatives have been discussed. Finally the arrangements for post-operative care should be discussed and recorded in the notes. It should be clear that the patient is aware that they must be accompanied home and that there should be a responsible adult with them until the following day, and that they are able to get help and return them in the event of any complications. Obviously they should not drive a vehicle for at least two days afterwards.

It is normal for the patient to be seen by an anaesthetist after their initial consultation or alternatively an appropriately trained nurse who will do an anaesthetic assessment on the anaesthetist's behalf.

Patients should have an empty stomach while anaesthetised; this is to reduce the chance of them regurgitating food and inhaling stomach contents while their normal reflexes are compromised. They should be informed of the local food and fluids policy which normally limits food intake for six hours beforehand and drink for two. Clear fluids and medication is usually permitted but not chewing gum as this stimulates salivary secretion. Policy sometimes varies between institutions so you need to check local policy.

The Anaesthetic process

We will mention the purely inhalation anaesthetic for dental extraction which used to be the norm and is now largely abandoned. However you may find that it is still used in some facilities to provide rapid anaesthesia of a short duration for simple dental extraction for children.

Here the patient was anaesthetised by inhalation of a gaseous mixture of nitrous oxide and oxygen through a mask designed to fit over the nose. This was often supplemented with a volatile anaesthetic gas. Traditionally the technique was used in the dental chair and often involved the patient being given up to 80% nitrous oxide with 20% oxygen at induction so that they were hypoxic for part of the time. The main advantage of this technique was that it was quick and cheap and many children could have their decayed teeth removed in one session. The main disadvantage for the surgeon was that they had a very limited time to operate. It was OK for a few deciduous or periodontally involved teeth but if roots were snapped off, they had to be left behind as there was no time to do a surgical procedure.

With this technique the surgeon was sharing the airway with the anaesthetist; they had to place swabs in the back of the

---

Pre-anaesthetic Food & Drink Policy:

May vary slightly between institutions

- No food from 6 hours before anaesthetic
- Milky, fizzy or fresh fruit drinks as for food
- Clear fluids encouraged up to 2 hours before
- Avoid chewing gum

Medication:

Anaesthetist or pre-assessment nurse may give specific instructions but generally:

- Regular medication should be taken with 50 mls. water
- Oral hypoglycemics should be omitted and the hospital protocol for diabetics followed

---

mouth and have good assistance with suction to prevent blood, saliva or tooth fragments from getting into the pharynx and being inhaled. However this hardly ever happened and the technique was generally safe as the patient was never deeply anaesthetised and it was rapid.

Now most oral surgery under general anaesthetic will be done on what is referred to as a 'day stay' or 'ambulatory' basis where the patient will come into the hospital for a day or half day.

On arrival before the beginning of the operating session the patient will be checked by a nurse; if it is a child the nurse will have had paediatric training. They will go through the medical and medication history again, check that they are appropriately starved and accompanied; they will be weighed and ASA graded. The patient will be seen by the anaesthetist and the anaesthetic explained. The surgeon will check the medical history, examine the surgical site, reiterate warnings, reconfirm their consent and ask if they have any questions not previously answered.

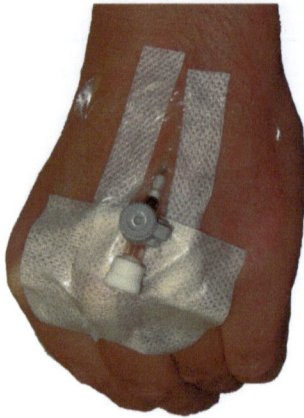

An intravenous cannula is placed (usually in the back of the hand) to give IV induction or use administer drugs in an emergency

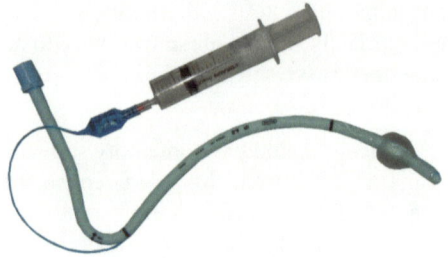

Nasal endotracheal tube. The anaesthetist passes the end of the tube through the vocal cords into the trachea then inflates the cuff with air from a syringe which seals the airway which helps prevent debris entering the trachea and helps secure it.

In the operating facility the patient will have an intravenous cannula inserted into a vein, usually in the back of the hand, and if it is a child this will have been preceded by local anaesthetic paste placed onto the cannulation site. Children are usually accompanied by a parent up to the stage when anaesthesia is induced when they leave.

Anaesthesia is usually induced with an intravenous agent such as propofol but a gaseous induction can be used with nitrous oxide and oxygen supplemented with a halogenated ether anaesthetic such as sevoflurane. Once anaesthesia is induced a breathing tube is placed; this may be an endotracheal tube placed through the mouth or nose into the trachea; the patient will breathe through this during the surgery and anaesthesia can be maintained with an anaesthetic, such as sevoflurane, added to the nitrous oxide/oxygen mixture or it can be maintained with an intravenous agent typically propofol.

To insert an endotracheal tube through the larynx the patient will need to either be quite deeply anaesthetised or given a drug to paralyse them. Generally it is easier for the anaesthetist to place an oral rather than a nasal tube but slightly less convenient for the surgeon as he will have to operate

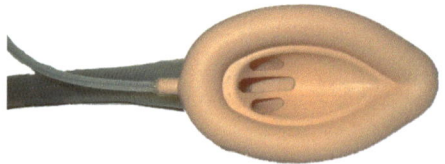

A laryngeal mask airway. Note that the tube is too thick to pass through the nasal cavities and must go through the mouth and is more difficult to work around than the thinner endotracheal tube.

around the tube. For a few cases such as removing or exposing impacted canines in the palate a nasal tube will be preferred.

The need to paralyse or give a deep anaesthetic can be obviated by use of a laryngeal mask airway which fits over the larynx to form a seal for the patient to breathe through. This makes everything quicker but from the surgeon's point of view the tube through the mouth is wider and therefore inconvenient to work around and from the anaesthetist's point of view it is likely to be disturbed by the surgeon who may have to stop while it is re-sited. Once the tube is placed the anaesthetist will place a pack in the pharynx to catch any blood, saliva or tooth fragments from the mouth.

This technique means that the airway of the patient is controlled and there is no risk of inhalation of debris. The patient will be monitored with a pulse oximeter for oxygen saturation and pulse rate, a blood pressure cuff for blood pressure and an ECG tracing for cardiac activity. The readings will be displayed onto a screen on the anaesthetic machine and there will be a monitor in the breathing circuit to measure exhaled carbon dioxide concentration.

Throughout, the surgeon should keep the anaesthetist informed of the progress and at the end, they should place a pack over the alveolus for the patient to bite on – which aids haemostasis – remove the throat pack and suck out the pharynx. Normally the anaesthetist will use a laryngoscope to examine down to the larynx to ensure it is clear. Once satisfied an oral airway is passed through the mouth so that breathing cannot be obstructed by the tongue and the patient delivered to the recovery area where their recovery will be supervised by a recovery nurse who will remove the oral airway when the patient is able to cough, and the pack 20 minutes or so later.

The patient is kept in the recovery area until they have been seen by the anaesthetist who will give permission for them to leave. The patient's welfare remains the responsibility of the anaesthetist until they have left recovery.

The patient will normally remain in the hospital day care facility until seen again at the end of the session by the surgeon and anaesthetist. Before they go they should be given verbal and written instructions, including how to make contact in the event of complications or anxieties. It is not normal to offer routine follow up appointments for dental extractions, simple or otherwise.

Suggested post-operative instructions:

• Be accompanied home by an adult

• Rest at home

• No driving for 48 hours

• Avoid any activity requiring judgement. Such as:

  Operating equipment
  Looking after small children alone
  Signing legal documents
  Social media
  Internet shopping

Examination tip:

▪ Be prepared to explain to a 'patient' (actor) the procedure they will go through to have a general anaesthetic for minor oral surgery and give them pre-anaesthetic instructions.

17 Spreading Dental Infection

Nearly all patients who present to oral and maxillofacial surgery departments in need of hospital admission for spreading dental infection have previously been seen by a health care professional and had inadequate management of a dental abscess; usually antibiotics alone. Usually they have seen a dentist but often a medical practitioner because they have been unable to find a dentist who would help them. Doctors are unable to do anything to help but prescribe antibiotics.

Whenever a diagnosis of an acute periapical abscess is made it must be treated by drainage. This is achieved either by opening the tooth with an air turbine drill to drain it, removing the tooth or if there is a fluctuant swelling, which suggests the presence of pus, then it should be incised. The management of a dental abscess with antibiotics alone is never acceptable.

If the tooth is opened through the root canal for pus to drain and not sealed the root canal will become colonised with oral flora making subsequent endodontic treatment more difficult, but it must not be sealed if there is still pus draining; the primary objective is to drain the pus and prevent infection spreading. However in most cases where there is that much pus the tooth will probably need removing anyway.

If the tooth is beyond subsequent restoration then it should be extracted. However the presence of pus can compromise achieving good local anaesthesia. If this becomes a problem then a nerve block followed by infiltration around the swelling may be successful. If necessary local anaesthetic must be injected into the infected area; the concern that this will spread infection and make the clinical situation worse is theoretical and outdated. The optimal treatment is to remove the cause and allow drainage. Giving the patient antibiotics and leaving pus undrained with

---

Dental Abscess History Checklist

• Site, duration, nature and any radiation of pain
• Sensitivity to hot, cold pressure, chewing
• History of any swelling or bad taste
• Past medical history and medication
• Past dental history & recent treatment
• Limitation of mouth opening

Dental Abscess Examination

• Caries, periodontal disease
• Teeth tender to percussion or lateral mobility
• Intra oral swelling or discharging sinus
• Pulp testing or sensitivity to cold (in some cases)
• Restriction of mouth opening or lateral movement
• Extra oral swelling and consistency, tenderness
• Cervical lymphadenopathy
• Temperature (in some cases)

---

the causative tooth in situ is the best way of allowing the abscess to flourish.

In nearly all cases drainage and/or tooth removal will be all the immediate treatment needed for an acute dental abscess. However in some cases it will be appropriate to prescribe antibiotics as well. This will be where the pus has penetrated through the periosteum and there is a spreading cellulitis through the soft tissues, the patient is systemically unwell, as indicated by pyrexia, or is immunocompromised. If there is a soft swelling of short duration then this may indicate inflammatory oedema alone rather than a collection of pus then treatment may not necessarily be so radical.

Most dental abscesses contain a mixture of organisms from the normal oral flora and the constituents vary as the abscess matures.

These comprise anaerobic Gram +ve cocci and Gram-ve rods with facultative anaerobic organisms. In the few occasions where antibiotics are indicated amoxicillin and metronidazole combined are adequate with erythromycin substituted for the amoxicillin in patients allergic to penicillin. Treatment should not be extended to beyond three days without reviewing the situation as longer courses lead to the emergence of resistant species. Antibiotics must never be used for chronic abscess.

Where pus is drained it is accepted practice for a swab of the pus to be sent for microbiological analysis to ascertain the causative organisms and their antibiotic sensitivity. However for dental abscesses there is little evidence that this makes any difference to the clinical outcome in otherwise fit patients. Most abscesses will be treated successfully with drainage and either extraction or endodontic management without antibiotics so antibiotic sensitivity is irrelevant. The patients are usually significantly improved by the time results are back from a microbiology laboratory.

Pus consists of living and dead bacteria, inflammatory cells, particularly polymorphs, inflammatory fluid, bacterial exotoxins and tissue debris. It will spread through the tissues along the least resistance. If the masticatory muscles are involved then mouth opening may be limited and a significant release of toxins into the blood stream will cause the patient to be pyrexial. Both of these events suggest a serious infection and referral to hospital will probably be indicated.

In severe cases pus may spread into the sublingual, buccal, submandibular or pterygomandibular spaces. In some severe cases the patient will need hospital admission. Usually intravenous antibiotics are used to localise a spreading infection and then surgery to remove the causative teeth and extra oral drainage.

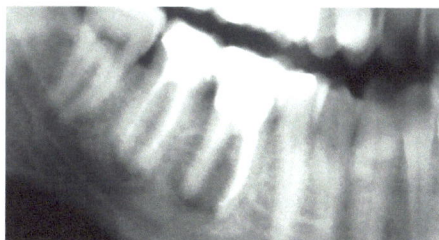

This patient reported no pain from the chronic infection related to the distal root of the non vital lower 6

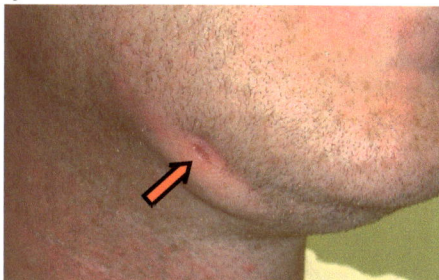

It was discharging below the mandible; therefore no build up of pressure

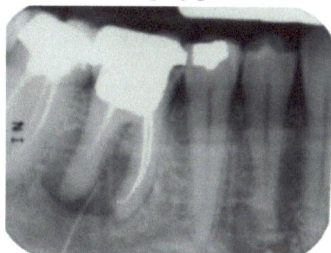

A periapical X-ray with a GP point in the sinus shows it leads to the apical lucency

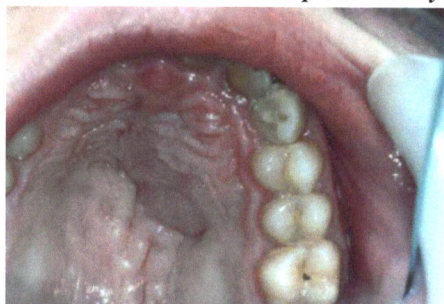

Acute abscess from upper canine. The palate is swollen and it is painful; drainage and removal of the tooth are both needed.

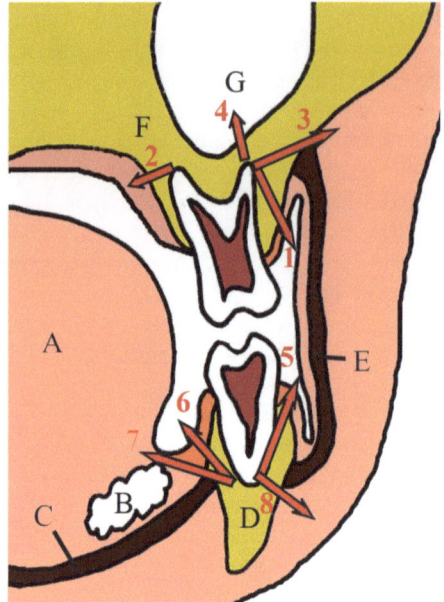

Spread of Infection from the Teeth:

Upper

1. Through alveolus to buccal sulcus (most common)

2. Through to palatal soft tissue (less common)

3. Above buccinator to buccal space

4. Into antrum (unusual)

Lower

5. Through alveolus to buccal sulcus (most common)

6. Through lingual bone into sublingual tissues

7. Through lingual bone into mouth (rare)

8. Buccally beneath buccinator to buccal space

Infection from lower molars can also track backwards behind the mylohyoid muscle to pterygomandibular space and down into submandibular space to neck

A: tongue B: sublingual gland C: mylohyoid muscle D: mandible E: buccinator F: maxilla G: antrum

It is unusual for a dental abscess to lead to death but it can happen, particularly in Ludwig's angina where a dental infection forms pus bilaterally in the floor of the mouth. Many of these cases have a pre-existing immunocompromising disease.

Indications for Hospital Admission

- Large facial swelling
- Firm facial swelling
- Cervical lymphadenopathy
- Trismus
- Difficulty swallowing
- Inability to eat or drink
- Pyrexia

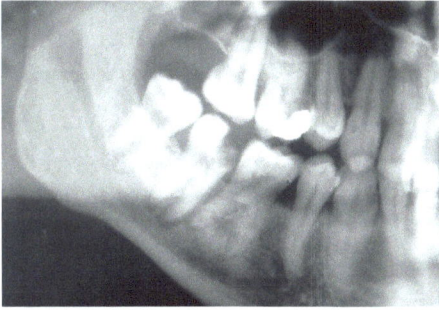

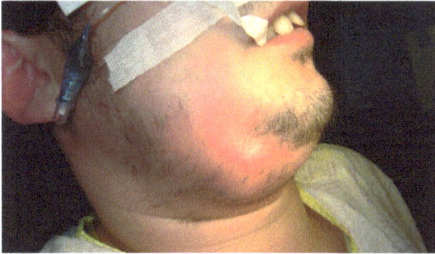

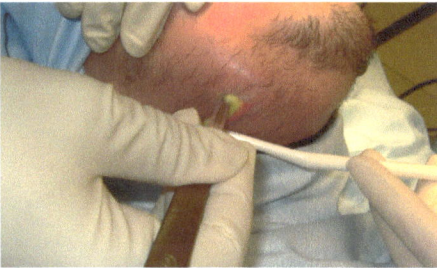

A submandibular abscess from lower right second molar. The pus had tracked behind the mylohyoid muscle into the submandibular space and now needs draining extra-orally. The patient went to the dentist but was just given antibiotics so it has exacerbated to this.

Quite a large variety of non malignant soft tissue lesions may present to us for surgical management but only a small number of these are common. All lesions should have a diagnosis made and usually this will involve a biopsy for histological confirmation of a provisional diagnosis. Here we will discuss the commoner soft tissue lesions in the mouth which may benefit from surgery.

Fibrous Hyperplasia

This is probably the commonest benign soft tissue swelling in the mouth. Here the soft tissues are scarred as a result of trauma and as a result of the swelling they can become more traumatised and increase to a great size. Most commonly this is seen on the buccal mucosa in line with the occlusal plane as a fibro-epithelial polyp catching between the teeth; less commonly this can occur on the tongue. These lesions can easily be removed with local anaesthetic.

Denture hyperplasia is fibrous hyperplasia caused by denture movement. If the patient leaves the denture out for some time the tissue will regress and then a smaller remnant can be removed surgically with care taken to avoid reducing the sulcus depth. However patients are usually reluctant to leave dentures out and now it is more usual to remove the tissue with a laser or cutting diathermy which will control bleeding as the surgery progresses.

Gingival overgrowths

Most gingival swellings are related to accumulation of dental calculus and plaque but there are several which are not related to chronic periodontal disease and require removal.

A peripheral giant cell granuloma or epulis is the commonest benign soft tissue swelling after the fibro-epithelial polyp; it usually occurs between teeth in the anterior mouth. It contains giant cells and blood

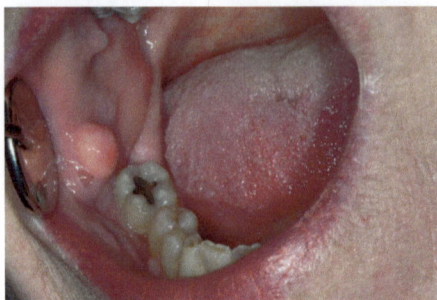

Fibro-epithelial polyp. The patient noticed this a few weeks beforehand. It was becoming a considerable nuisance as he was catching it between his teeth when eating. It was easily removed surgically.

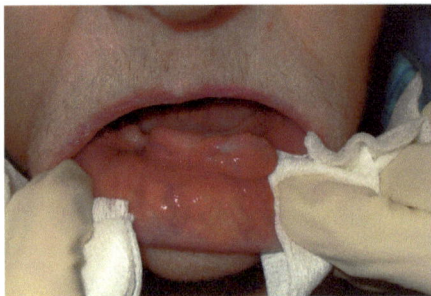

Denture hyperplasia. This was removed with a CO_2 laser so the patient was able to use her denture while it healed before replacement.

vessels and tends to have a blue/purple tinge; it should be removed with a small margin and the base curetted to discourage recurrence. The word peripheral is used to distinguish it from the rare central giant cell granuloma arising within the jaws.

The pyogenic granuloma is normally pedunculated and consists of granulation tissue and many blood vessels so that it is soft and oedematous and bleeds easily. It results from local irritation and can occur on the skin as well as within the mouth and is particularly common in children; the lesion should be removed with a small margin of normal tissue and can recur if this is not done.

A pregnancy epulis is similar histologically; it is a localised lesion found

Benign Soft Tissue Lesions

Commoner:

Fibrous Hyperplasia: Fibro-epithelial polyp and denture hyperplasia, caused by local trauma

Peripheral Giant Cell Granuloma: Anterior mouth between the teeth, has blue/purple tinge and bleeds easily

Pyogenic Granuloma: Usually pedunculated, bleeds easily, can occur on skin

Pregnancy Epulis: An exaggerated response to plaque in pregnancy, may be localised or more general, similar histology to pyogenic granuloma

Fibrous Epulis: A firmer epulis, histologically like fibrous hyperplasia but between the teeth

Drug Induced Gingival Hyperplasia: Most commonly from phenytoin, calcium channel blockers and ciclosporin

High frenal attachments: Lingual or labial, usually surgery not needed

Salivary Swellings: chapter 22

Less Common:

Papillomas: viral warts, may be sexually transmitted, suspect immunosuppression if present in large numbers

Haemangiomas: Vary from small degenerative haemangiomas in the lip of the elderly (common) to large proliferative haemangiomas which are potentially dangerous and rare

Palatal tumours: Usually a benign tumour of minor salivary glands (usually pleomorphic adenoma) or less frequently lymphoma

Diffuse Sub-mucosal Swelling: Orofacial granulomatosis (particularly lips), Crohns's, sarcoidosis (rare)

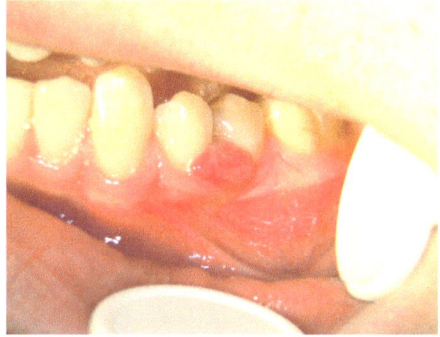

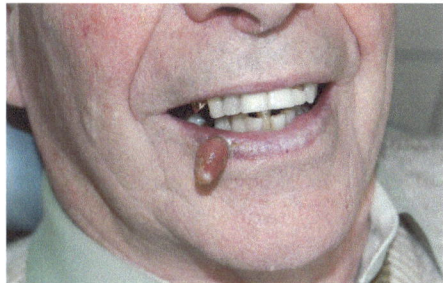

Pyogenic granulomas

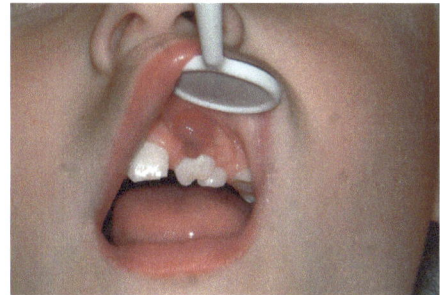

Peripheral giant cell granuloma. It was prone to bleed when traumatised

during pregnancy which usually resolves, at least partly, after the child is born. It is probably due to hormonal changes in the response to plaque and unless the lesion bleeds profusely it should be reviewed post-partum when no surgery may be needed. Occasionally these lesions may be more generalised or diffuse.

The fibrous epulis is another variation of fibrous hyperplasia which usually arises between teeth and, like the fibro-epithelial polyp, will be firm with the consistency of rubber. It too results from local trauma but may be exacerbated by poor plaque control and become inflamed. It may be sessile or

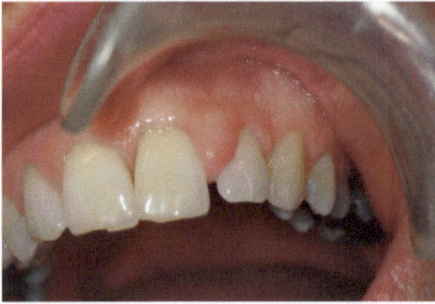

A fibrous epulis. They may be pedunculated or sessile like this one; it is firmish with the consistancy of rubber and does not readily bleed when probed

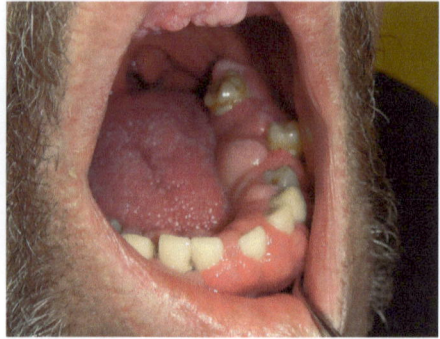

Gingival hyperplasia in this case caused by ciclosporin used to prevent rejection of a kidney transplant. It may best be removed surgically with a cutting diathermy which will also control the inevitable bleeding. A carbon dioxide laser is best avoided as it may mark the enamel. Recurrence is likely but may be delayed by meticulous oral hygiene but the medication should not be stopped as the patient will need his transplanted kidney more than he doesn't need the hyperplasia

pedunculated and should be surgically excised with a small margin of normal tissue and the bed of the wound curetted. Occasionally calcified tissue may be formed within it.

Gingival swelling can be caused as a side effect of a number of drugs, most commonly phenytoin used for epilepsy; calcium channel blocker used for heart disease, particularly hypertension; and ciclosporin, an immunosuppressant used in organ transplantation.

Tongue tie

Many children are born with a lingual frenum attached to the crest of the mandibular alveolus, or nearly so. Some may be referred by a midwife or health visitor as a matter of course for frenectomy. The request to carry out surgery should be resisted unless there is an obvious problem. The problems alleged to be caused are difficulty with breast feeding and interference with phonating certain sounds when speech develops after 14 months of age. In the majority of cases as the alveolus develops during growth the frenal attachment will migrate comparatively downwards and the child will have no permanent problem. Some will not progress in this manner and the high attachment may compromise oral hygiene or lead to periodontal breakdown when the patient is older. These cases will benefit from frenectomy; surgery will be very minor and

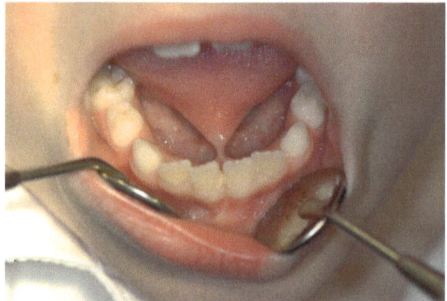

Tongue tie compromising oral hygiene

swiftly carried out with local anaesthetic. In the meantime some mothers may present complaining that the limitation of tongue movement is hindering feeding or speech development. In these circumstances it is prudent to operate on the basis that mothers are usually right. We have no reliable scientific evidence.

In a few cases a low labial frenum may be attached to the crest of the maxillary alveolus and preventing a mid-line diastema from closing. In this case frenectomy may be indicated, taking care to remove the fibrous attachment between the incisors. This should only be done in conjunction with an orthodontist. It is normally done just before they close the space; otherwise it may well just recur.

Papillomas

Oral warts or squamous cell papillomas are caused by several of the human papilloma virus sub-types, including the ones associated with sexual transmission. They may be transmitted sexually or not. They are of low infectivity and may be spread among families or children from their fingers. They may persist with no virus present. They commonly occur singly or as a small number and can be removed surgically taking a small margin of normal tissue or treated with cryotherapy; this is usually curative. If they are present in large numbers it suggests immunosuppression, most particularly HIV. This is unusual now as triple therapy for HIV infection usually cures the problem. They should not be removed with a laser as the resulting smoke has been known to transmit papillomas to the larynx of the operator.

Haemangiomas

Large arteriovenous malformations or proliferative haemangiomas which may risk bleeding should be referred to a specialist team for management which may include embolization before surgery. However a large number of smaller cavernous haemangiomas may be seen in the mouth, many of which require no active treatment at all. Many in children will regress with age but a good number of unsightly lesions are seen, particularly in the lips of older persons, which may be managed successfully with laser treatment or cryotherapy.

Palatal Swellings

The most common swelling of the palate, other than acute swelling of a dental abscess, is a pleomorphic adenoma, a tumour of salivary tissue. These are benign but must be removed with a wide margin to prevent recurrence and will best be done

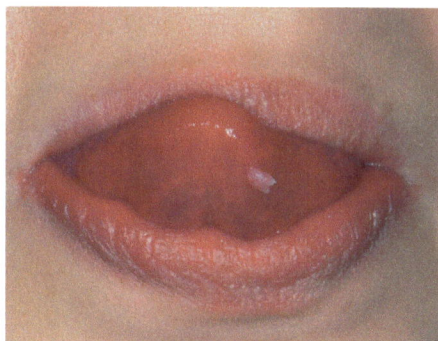

Viral papilloma

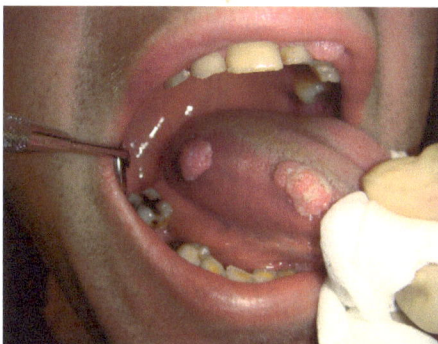

Multiple viral papillomas

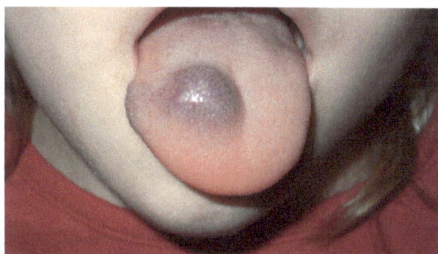

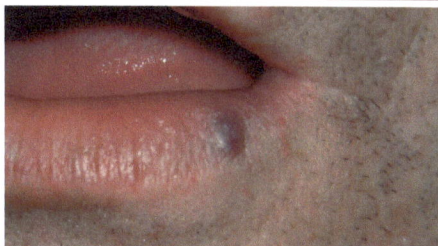

Haemangiomas. The ones on the lip are particularly common in older age

in hospital under anaesthetic in order to facilitate the radical surgery needed. Lymphomas may also occur in the palate. A large biopsy will be required for the pathologist to examine the architecture for diagnosis and the patient should be referred to the lymphoma team for management. In the palate the lesion is likely to be a MALT (mucosa associated lymphoid tissue) lymphoma which particularly occurs in patients with Sjogren's syndrome and is of very low grade malignancy.

Diffuse sub-mucosal swelling

Diffuse swelling beneath the mucosa may be due to chronic granulomatous disease. Orofacial granulomatosis (OFG) may be seen particularly in young adults. Submucosal swelling may be accompanied by angular stomatitis and cracking of the lips; the mucosa is frequently described as having a cobble-stone appearance. The lesion should be biopsied and the patient may be investigated for Crohn's disease if they give no history of it, as a small number may present with identical mouth lesions.

OFG may be caused by some sort of allergy so the management is not surgical. Sarcoidosis may produce granulomatous oral swellings; the patients should be examined and investigated for salivary and lymph node swelling, particularly the hilar nodes in the chest. Many will be asymptomatic and require no treatment.

Benign tumours

There are a variety of benign tumours which can occur in the mouth and diagnosis has to be by excision biopsy and histological examination. Generally they tend to be rarer than the conditions mentioned hitherto. Dentists should be aware that neurofibromas can occur in the mouth. They may be solitary but often they will be part of neurofibromatosis type 1 which is a genetic disease which is autosomal dominant with frequent new mutations and is one of the more common genetic disorders. Patients often have many of these tumours and most have some in the mouth where they may present. They are usually accompanied by pigmented lesions on the skin, café au lait spots.

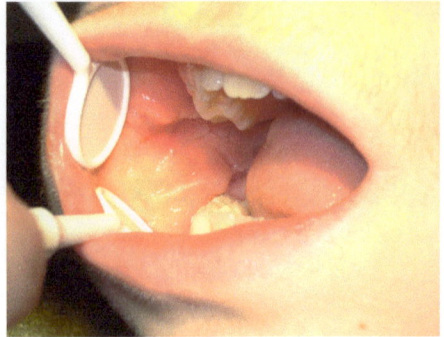

This nobbly appearance of the oral mucosa in this child was diagnosed as oro-facial granulomatosis by biopsy. There were no other manifestations and no evidence of Crohn's disease

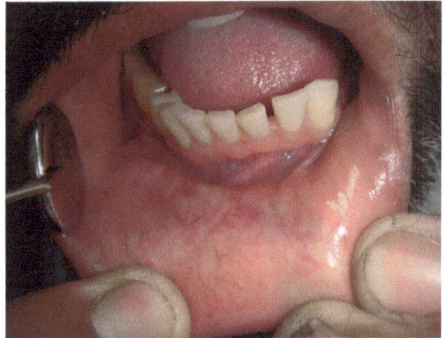

This swelling was caused by the granulomas of sarcoidosis. Chest X-ray showed enlargement of the hilar lymph nodes but the patient was asymptomatic so no active treatment was required

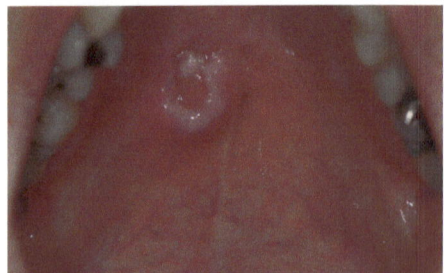

A benign tumour on the palate; most commonly these are pleomorphic salivary adenomas as this was. A large wide excision is required

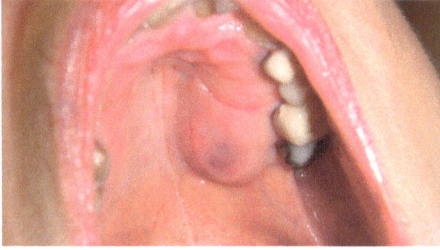

A MALT lymphoma on palate

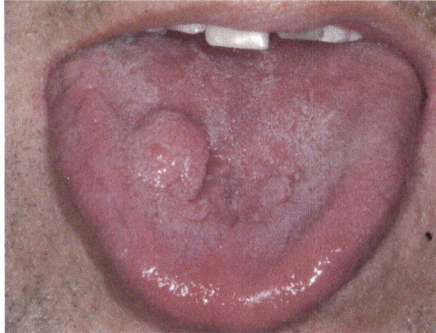

Neurofibroma of tongue. This may be a solitary lesion; look for other lesions in the mouth or beneath the skin and café au lait skin marks. Their presence indicates neurofibromatosis type 1

19 Oral Cancer and its Natural History

The most common cancer affecting the mouth is the squamous cell carcinoma. It is likely that most dentists working in primary care will see only a few in their careers but missing one can be catastrophic for the patient; the earlier it is diagnosed and treated the better the prognosis. Overall about half of patients survive their oral squamous cancers, although with a higher risk of developing another cancer somewhere in the upper aero-digestive tract.

To recognise these cancers it is helpful to have seen some before so you should seize any opportunity you can to go to clinics where they are assessed. You should take histories from the patients, examine the tumours, including feeling them with a gloved finger.

Squamous cancer arises from the stratified squamous epithelium of the mouth. It may arise from within a 'potential malignant condition' particularly when there is dysplasia present but usually it arises de novo. Dysplasia indicates a heightening risk, not a certainty, of a cancer developing and the absence of dysplasia does not mean no cancer will develop. We do not know exactly what the aetiology is but we do know that there are risk factors, some of which are self-inflicted, such as smoking, high alcohol intake and paan chewing (betel leaf, tobacco, slaked lime and areca nut) and others which are not, such as increasing age.

Initially an early lesion is asymptomatic. It is possible that some microscopic lesions will be controlled by the patient's immunity but they may eventually grow and infiltrate the surrounding tissues and ulcerate through the mucous membrane. As the lesion enlarges and involves nervous tissue or becomes infected it will become painful and this is when the patient normally seeks help unless a dentist has already noticed something untoward and referred them for investigation.

The lesions will continue to increase in size and infiltrate the tissues with some patients not presenting for investigation until the tumour has reached a considerable size. Eventually there will be spread to the lymph glands in the neck. The spread will usually be sequentially down the neck but some tongue cancers may skip some of the nodes and initially metastasize lower down.

Oral squamous cancer is usually slow to metastasize to distant sites in the body

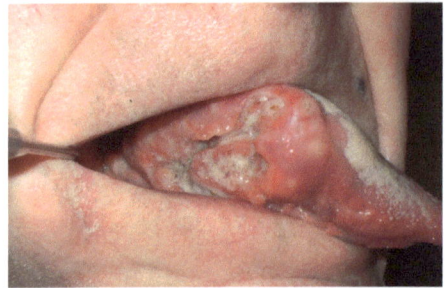

A large squamous cancer on the side of a tongue. Note the typical raised rolled margin and the slough in the ulcer. It feels hard when palpated and will bleed easily if manipulated. It is painful and smells

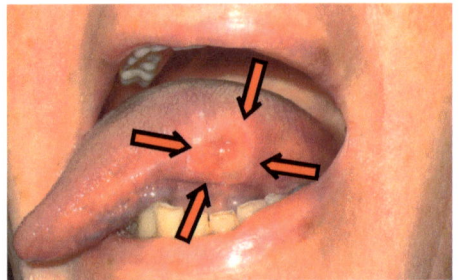

An early squamous cancer. It has just started to become sore, it is firm to palpate and the patient was rightly becoming anxious. Generally the smaller the tumour at presentation the better the prognosis. However each tumour has its own (abnormal) genetic make-up, hence its own character and they behave differently. Tongue tumours in particular can be unpredictable with some small ones being very nasty and larger ones less unpleasant than they initially look

but they can do so. Death can occur from distant metastases but is more usually from recurrence at the primary site or in the neck. Unlike some tumours such as bronchial carcinoma, where a weakened cachectic patient slowly fades and dies peacefully from bronchopneumonia, the oral cancer patient dies from asphyxiation or bleeding from the recurrence in mouth or neck.

Patients should have their neck glands palpated, their mouth fully examined and the suspicious lesion examined, measured with a ruler and palpated. The typical lesion will have a ragged, indurated, raised margin, will be tender to palpate and hard. There will often be a characteristic smell as it will be infected and when biopsied the scalpel blade has a characteristic feel of being like sand embedded in butter; the tissue will tear and fragment easily.

If you see a patient with a suspicious lesion in dental practice you should refer them to hospital without delay. In NHS hospitals there will a system to refer potentially malignant lesions so that they are seen with a guarantee of being seen within two weeks of referral. You should always know what the system is; it usually involves the patient being referred to a central administrator who will make sure that the patient sees an appropriate clinician within the target of 14 days; their progress will then be tracked. Sending a letter to the local consultant usually won't do; the patient will not then be in the 'cancer' referral 'pathway' and their progress will not be 'tracked' and monitored. Do not biopsy yourself but make sure that any written referral has the words 'suspected cancer' in it and that the patient knows your concern. It is important that they understand and do not delay an appointment.

In our experience most delays in referral have been related to lesions on the lateral border of the tongue which were not taken seriously enough. An apparently small area of mucosal damage caused by dental trauma can be mimicked by a small invasive cancer. Dental trauma must be observed to

---

Dysplasia

Grading

Is Mild, Moderate or Severe, but the grading is inexact

Grading depends on architecture of epithelium:

Irregular stratification, loss of polarity of basal cells, drop-shaped rete ridges, increased mitotic figures, abnormal superficial mitoses and keratin pearls in rete ridges

Grading also depends on cell atypia:

Variation in cell size and shape, nucleus size

Shape and number and atypical mitotic figures.

---

heal completely (not just improved) after removal of the apparent cause before a patient may be reassured and discharged from follow up.

Oral squamous cancer will be treated by a head and neck cancer multidisciplinary team which will have oral & maxillofacial, ENT and sometimes plastic surgeons as well as an oncologist and pathologist as core members. Treatment depends upon the patient and the stage at presentation but mostly it will consist of surgery which may be followed by radiotherapy.

Large lesions may be shrunk with combined chemotherapy and radiotherapy at the start. It is essential that all patients with oral, nasal or pharyngeal tumours should have a comprehensive assessment of their dentition as soon as they are diagnosed so that they are rendered dentally fit before treatment starts. In most centres the patients are assessed by a restorative dentist which will give the patient the opportunity to discuss future prosthetic rehabilitation.

There has been an increase in oro-pharyngeal cancer (base of tongue, tonsil and pharynx) related to Human Papilloma Virus which particularly occurs in younger,

Features of malignant & benign tumours compared	
Malignant	**Benign**
Infiltrates local tissues	Displaces local tissues
Irregular ill defined margin	Well defined circumscribed margin
Spreads through lymphatics and blood to distant sites	Enlarges locally but does spread elsewhere
Painful except when quite small	Usually painless
Untreated causes death	Untreated reaches enormous size with symptoms only arising from pressure e.g. intracranially can cause death from brain compression

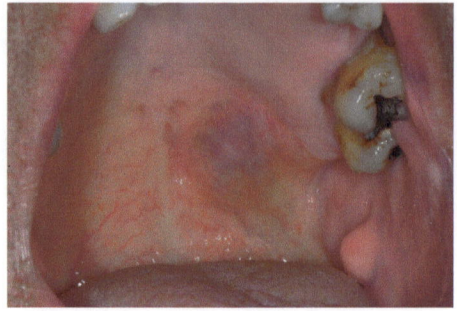

Adenocystic carcinoma from minor salivary gland in palate

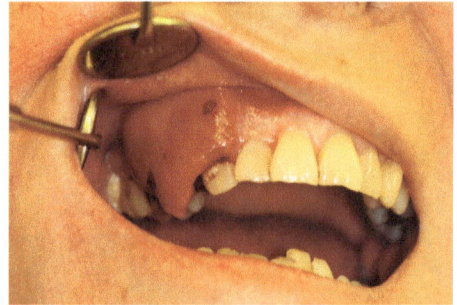

A b-cell lymphoma on the alveolus

otherwise healthier, patients whose condition is unrelated to smoking or a high alcohol intake. These cases usually have a better prognosis and are often treated using chemo-radiotherapy without surgery. The virus is the same as that causing cervical cancer and when the population has been adequately immunised against the virus these oral cancers should cease.

In addition to the oral squamous cell carcinoma which is the most common cancer of the mouth there are several others which although not rare are less usual. Several of these come from minor salivary glands which are situated beneath the mucosa all around the mouth but particularly in the palate. Among these are the mucoepidermoid carcinomas which exhibit a spectrum of behaviour from being almost benign to nasty like squamous cell carcinomas and adenocystic carcinomas which when removed have a very high five years survival rate but infiltrate slowly along nerves and produce distant metastases many years after the patient has considered themselves cured. Polymorphous low grade adenocarcinomas are malignant and infiltrate but tend to have a very good prognosis and there is necrotising sialometaplasia which looks very malignant in appearance but which is not a tumour at all.

Very rarely a swelling may be caused by leukaemia and less uncommonly a lymphoma which may arise from lymph tissue embedded within the salivary glands. Sometimes lymphomas can arise from lymphoid tissue which is found in the mucosa in Sjorgren's syndrome (MALT - mucosa associated lymphoid tissue). Lymphomas are rubbery in consistency and MALT lymphomas are slow growing and easily treated with radiotherapy.

Very occasionally metastatic cancer from elsewhere in the body may be seen in the mouth. This may be from elsewhere in the gastro-intestinal tract but less unusually will metastasize to the mandible from kidney, lung, breast or prostate. There are also some rare odontogenic tumours in the jaws (see chapter 20).

The message here is that mouth malignancies can vary in appearance and every undiagnosed swelling or non healing ulcer should be referred to an oral & maxillofacial surgeon through the urgent 'two week referral' cancer service.

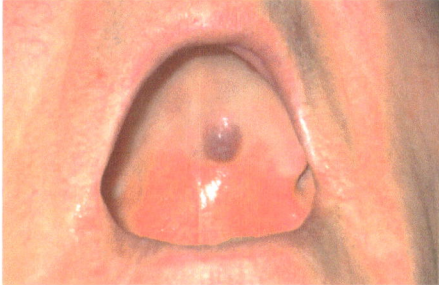

Adenocarcinoma from minor salivary gland in palate

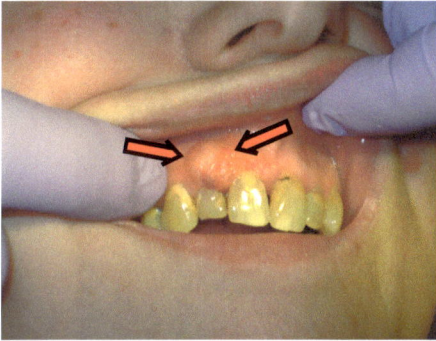

Keratinising squamous cell carcinoma on upper alveolus. This didn't look suspicious enough to be referred for some time so treatment was unnecessarily delayed. However it was slow growing and she was cured.

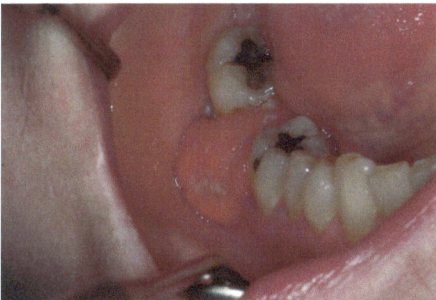

Squamous cell carcinoma on lower alveolus

Risk factors for oral squamous cell carcinoma	
Risk	**Note**
Previous squamous cancer in upper aero-digestive tract	
Advanced age	
Smoking	Also for many other cancers
High alcohol intake	When combined with smoking multiplies rather than adds to the risk
Paan chewing and sub-mucous fibrosis	On the buccal mucosa - which is an unusual site otherwise
Human papilloma virus	Usually at back of mouth posterior tongue, tonsils oro-pharynx

Examination tip:

- An understanding of mouth cancer diagnosis, its recognition, risk factors and potentially malignant conditions are rightly considered a priority by examiners in dental qualifying examinations.

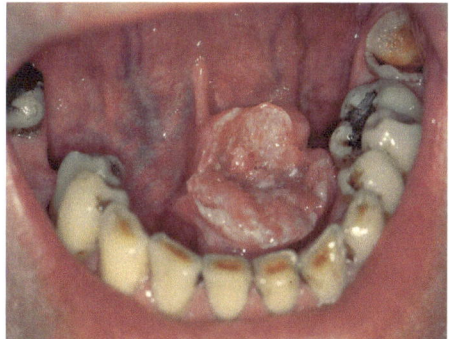

Squamous cell carcinoma floor of mouth

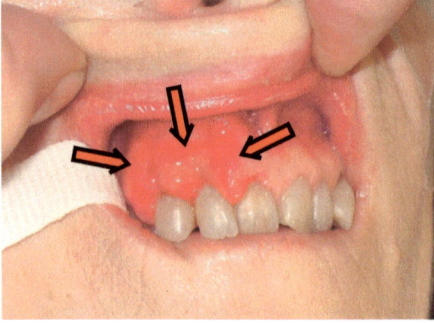

Spindle cell carcinoma on upper alveolus. Again referral was delayed for weeks while the dentist managed it with repeated antibiotics. It too was cured

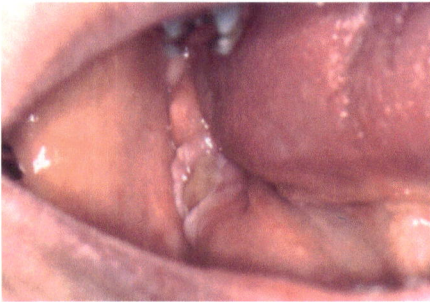

Not a cancer but looks suspiciously like one. It was a traumatic ulcer caused by the unopposed upper molar

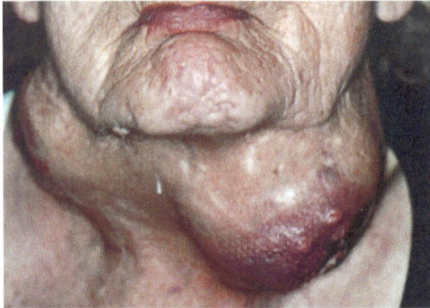

Metastatic lymph nodes from untreated oral squamous cancer. The patient moved house after her first hospital appointment and thought that if it was important she would be sent for. It was and she wasn't!

20 Odontogenic Cysts and Tumours

Odontogenic cysts are either inflammatory secondary to dental disease or developmental. We have listed these in the tables.

We do not think it necessary for you to be familiar with the behaviour of the rare odontogenic cysts or tumours for your clinical work or for non-specialist dental examinations. In the tables we have omitted the rarest ones which you are unlikely to see or be required to know about in your examinations.

However it is necessary to know that the commonest tumour ameloblastoma may present in the same way as an odontogenic cyst. These are benign and do not metastasize but they do invade locally. You should also know that the keratocyst behaves aggressively even though it is a cyst.

Most cysts present as a radiolucency on an x-ray image with a distinct dense periphery where the bone has reacted to the pressure of the expanding cyst. The other way of presenting is as an expansion of the alveolar bone and sometimes as an infection if the lesion has breached through the cortex and occasionally as a fracture of the mandible. You should always palpate to elicit any expansion of the bone, note any tooth movement and test for the vitality of adjacent teeth.

Odontogenic Inflammatory Cysts

Radicular: Most common; at apex of dead tooth; formed from epithelial rests in granuloma stimulated by inflammation from tooth, also includes the 'residual' cyst which is a radicular cyst which remains after the causative tooth is removed

Collateral Cysts: Rare 'paradental' cysts arising on lower third molars and lateral to 1st & 2nd molars. Uncertain aetiology

---

Odontogenic Developmental Cysts

Dentigerous Cyst: Next common to radicular; surrounds crown of unerupted tooth; most usually upper canine or lower third molar; forms from the dental follicle

Odontogenic Keratocyst: Has a very thin lining; thick cyst fluid containing keratin; usually multiloculated; wall has 'daughter cysts' and epithelial proliferation; high recurrence rate if parakeratinised lining; lower recurrence if orthokeratinised lining (rarer); tends not to expand cortex so spreads widely before presenting late; bony cavity should be curetted 1-2 mms to reduce recurrence

Lateral Periodontal Cyst: Lateral or between roots of a vital tooth; arises from odontogenic epithelial remnants

Eruption Cyst: Dentigerous cyst over crown of erupting tooth; ruptures as tooth erupts

Gingival Cyst: Arises from dental lamina rests; similar to lateral periodontal cyst; more common in infants where it resolves spontaneously; rare in adults where it needs removal

---

The most common will be a radicular cyst caused by dentally induced inflammation in a granuloma at the apex of a non-vital tooth. These will enlarge slowly over several years and eventually can reach a size large enough to penetrate the cortical bone and become infected, which is when the patient will present for treatment if they have not already been found from a routine dental x-ray. X-rays will show the lesion to be unilocular and there will be no resorption of the teeth. If the causative tooth or root has been removed the cyst will be called a residual cyst.

The second most common cyst is the developmental dentigerous cyst which occurs most commonly in the third molar region of the mandible and will be seen on

Benign Epithelial Odontogenic Tumours

Commoner:

Ameloblastoma: Locally aggressive; need surgical clearance of one cm; do not metastasise; large irregular bone cavity; expands cortical bone but it unusually penetrates through it; usually multiloculated, has a 'soap bubble' appearance on X-ray

Rarer:

Calcifying Epitheloid Odontogenic (Pindborg) Tumour: penetrates cancellous bone and expands cortex; does not penetrate cortex; may contain a tooth; behaves like ameloblastoma but can be mistaken for a malignancy; local excision with a margin of bone is adequate

Adenomatoid Odontogenic Tumour: Presents as a cyst which envelops the crown of a tooth

Squamous Odontogenic tumour: Consists of squamous epithelium which degenerates into cystic cavities; calcification may occur; can infiltrate cancellous bone and loosen teeth

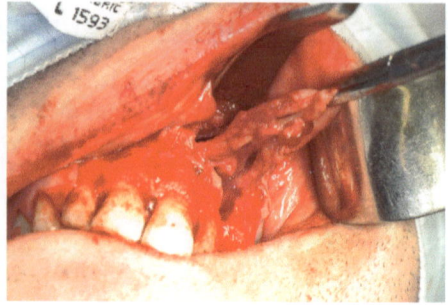

Operation to remove an apical cyst. The cyst fluid is thin and the lining thick and after loosening it with a curette it can be pulled out and the cavity curetted. A keratocyst would be more aggressive and contain a thick cyst fluid containing keratin but a thin friable lining which is more likely to recur

Benign Mixed Epithelial & Mesencymal Odontogenic Tumour

Ameloblastic fibroma: usually occurs in teens; slow growing & destructive; presents as a cyst; expands jaw; cured by complete removal

Odontoma: a hard tumour consisting of a bony matrix containing dentine and enamel

Benign Mesencymal Odontogenic Tumours

Odontogenic fibroma; a slow growing fibrous mass; usually in mandible; removal is usually easy and is curative

Odontogenic myxoma: occurs in the young; loose mucoid material infiltrates widely; should be removed with a wide margin; may recur years later

Cementoblastoma: usually seen in young; benign radiopacity at apex of mandibular molar surrounded by a lucency; should be removed with the tooth

x-ray as a radiolucent lesion enveloping the crown of an unerupted tooth.

It is normal for a provisional diagnosis to be made on the basis of the clinical and x-ray appearance. Standard treatment is surgical enucleation; the cyst is shelled out preferably without fragmenting it so as to improve the chance of leaving no part of the cyst lining behind. Smaller lesions, particularly in the anterior maxilla, can be removed with local anaesthesia, but larger lesions in areas where surgical access is more difficult are more usually done with general anaesthesia.

There are certain features of a cystic lesion which are suggestive of a keratocyst, ameloblastoma or one of the rarer odontogenic tumours which will need more radical treatment than a radicular or dentigerous cyst. These features are: rapid expansion of the cortical bone, large size, multi-locular appearance on the x-ray and loosening or resorption of the adjacent teeth.

Keratocysts may have small 'daughter cysts' arising from their linings; because of this and a higher mitotic activity in their linings they tend to recur. They must therefore be removed with a 1-2 mm margin of bone from around them. An ameloblastoma and some of the other odontogenic tumours may need a much more radical approach but not as radical as for an invasive cancer. However an ameloblastoma may initially be decompressed to reduce their size prior to surgical removal.

Marsupialisation is a technique used for very large cysts or for smaller lesions to avoid a more substantial operation in patients with medical co-morbidities; it can be done with local anaesthetic if in an

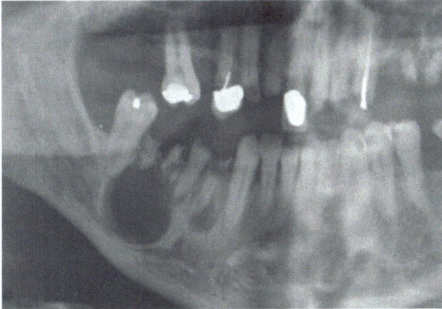

A radicular cyst related to the decayed roots

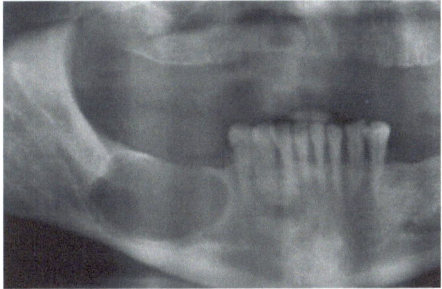

A residual cyst; the causative tooth has been previously removed

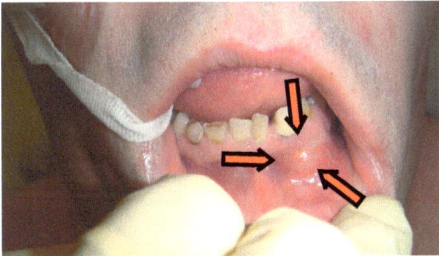

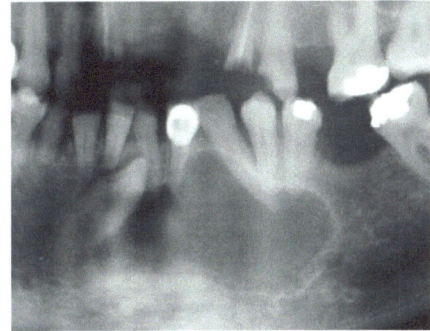

This radicular cyst presented with firm swelling of the labial sulcus. Had it not it would have eventually resorbed the labial bone and become infected

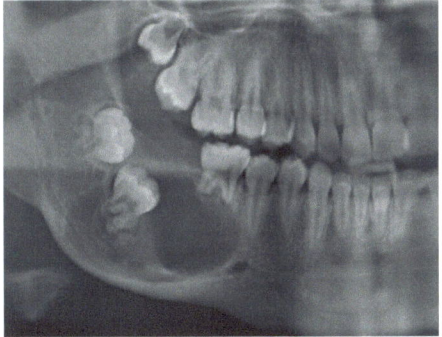

This lesion looks more aggressive from the x-ray appearance. Not only has the lower 7 been displaced but the root of the 6 has been eroded. This is an ameloblastoma. A radicular or residual cyst can be scraped out but this must be treated more radically with surrounding bone removal to prevent recurrence, but not as aggressively as a squamous cancer

accessible area of the mouth. This involves taking a window of bone and cyst lining but leaving the remainder of the lesion and so avoiding destroying bone or adjacent structures such as teeth or the inferior dental nerve. Again decompression may be used initially.

Some rarer non-odontogenic lesions such as ossifying fibroma, cemento-osseous dysplasia, and fibrous dysplasia can look cystic when they first start. If they are thought to be a cyst initially then it doesn't matter as they are benign. They just require more careful follow up after the surgery. Dentigerous or radicular cysts do not need to be followed up long term because they don't recur.

Examination tips:

- You should know the pathogenesis and management of the common dental cysts
- You should understand that odontogenic tumours may present in the same way as cysts and be able to explain a strategy for investigation and referral for management of suspected lesions
- A knowledge of all the rare odontogenic tumours and cysts is not essential for qualifying examinations. (Rare = those other than ameloblastoma and keratocyst)

21 <u>Non Odontogenic Jaw Swellings and Radiolucency</u>

The most common and significant bony jaw pathology concern of the dentist is MRONJ (Medication Related Osteonecrosis of the Jaw) Usually this will not cause problems until infection is introduced into the compromised bone by dental treatment, most typically extraction. Similarly bone damaged by radiotherapy is important but not normally an issue until dental extraction. These are both discussed in chapter 02.

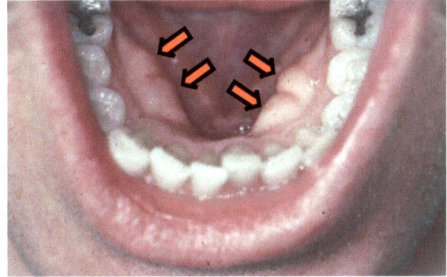

Mandibular tori. The patient discovered them and was worried

<u>Exostoses and Osteomas</u>

Maxillary and mandibular tori are benign bony swellings which form in adulthood and are located in the midline of the hard palate and lingual of the lower premolars respectively. Mandibular tori are normally bilateral. Patients may notice them after some time and be alarmed that they might have a tumour. The characteristic site and appearance is sufficient for you to reassure them of their benign nature and that no treatment is needed. However, occasionally the swellings may be a physical impediment to the wearing of prostheses, in which case they can be removed surgically.

Less commonly, bony exostoses may develop in other sites, often buccally in the maxilla and this may be a response to the inflammation of periodontal disease. These

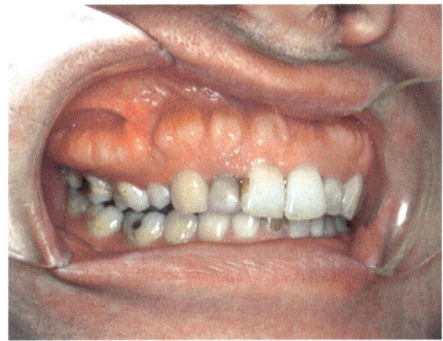

Benign maxillary exostoses

may be unsightly or prevent oral hygiene measures in which case they can be removed surgically. Rarely a benign osteoma may grow; this should be removed and subjected to histological examination to rule out a malignant sarcoma (which are rare). All these lesions if examined under the microscope will be identical i.e. dense bone.

<u>Fibro-osseous lesions</u>

The ossifying fibroma is the commonest non odontogenic jaw lesion comprising of fibrous tissue and bone. It usually occurs in the mandible and radiographically is well defined and has a mixed lucent and opaque appearance. The lesion should be removed surgically and the area comprehensively curetted. There is a more aggressive variant, juvenile aggressive ossifying fibroma, which will require resection with a margin of normal bone to control it and this variant may not

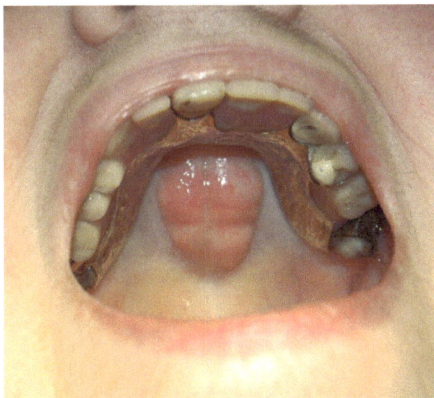

Palatal torus. The partial denture has been designed to avoid it

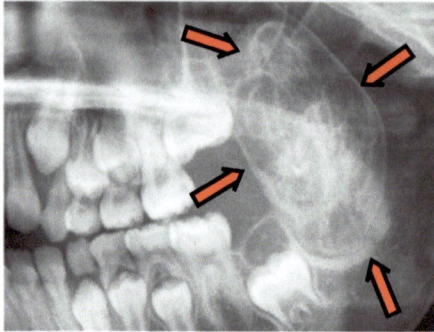

Ossifying fibroma

be easily distinguished by histology alone so must be followed up closely clinically and by imaging. In fact these lesions may represent a point on a spectrum towards osteosarcoma which is highly malignant but fortunately rare.

Fibrous dysplasia is caused by a genetic mutation and usually presents in the jaws as a painless swelling of the bone in childhood. The fibro-osseous process has a typical 'ground glass' appearance on X-ray. In most cases (about 70%) it occurs in one bone and in others in several as is known as the polyostotic variety. Usually it is self-limiting and no active treatment is needed. However, it may be reduced surgically if the facial appearance is compromised or it causes pressure symptoms on nerves.

Cherubism is an autosomal dominant genetic disorder causing fibro-osseous enlargement of the lower face in children and loss of deciduous teeth and mal-development of the permanent dentition. It usually aborts with increasing age. It is rare.

Cemento-osseous dysplasia is a fibro-osseous lesion seen most frequently in ladies of African descent in middle life often affecting the mandible; the lesion may be localised or affecting several areas. It may be asymptomatic and only discovered on routine X-ray or may cause swelling. The radiographic appearance is of radiolucent areas with opacities developing within them. The adjacent teeth are vital.

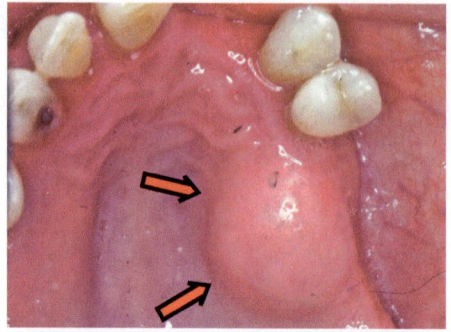

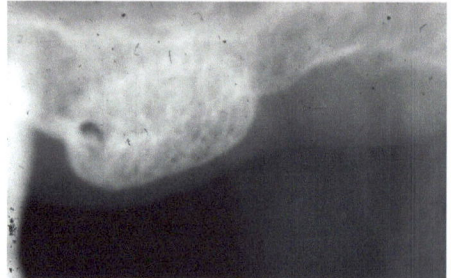

Osteoma on maxillary alveolus and its X-ray image

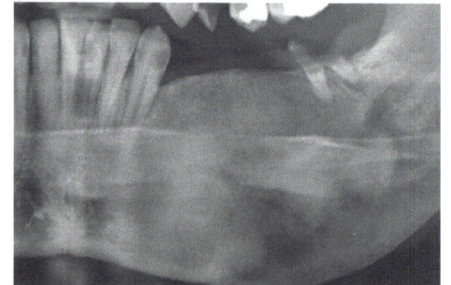

Fibrous dysplasia

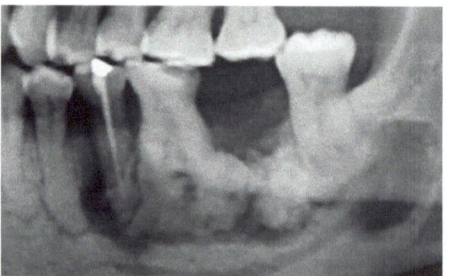

Cemento-osseous dysplasia

Cystic lesions

A naso-palatine duct cyst is normally seen as a chance finding on radiography It is formed from cells in the vestigial nasopalatine duct. It is seen as a

Commoner:

Palatal Torus: Harmless; only indication for removal is interference with denture wearing

Mandibular Tori: Harmless; only indication for removal is interference with denture wearing

Bony Exostoses: Harmless

Rarer:

Osteoma: Slow growing benign tumours of bone distinguished from the tori and exostoses only by their location

Ossifying fibroma: Slow growing fibro-osseous lesions containing collagen, bone or cementum. Be aware of the existence of the juvenile aggressive ossifying fibroma which is distinguished only by its behaviour

Central giant cell granuloma: usually young person central mandible

Nasopalatine duct cyst: heart shaped lucency +1 cm

Stafne's cyst: not a cyst; salivary tissue

Traumatic bone cyst: not a cyst; an empty space

Rare:

Fibrous dysplasia: Fibro-osseous lesion usually in young people, tends to be self limiting but can cause deformity and nerve compression

Cemento-osseous dysplasia: Affects mandible in 3rd & 4th decade usually in patients of African descent

Cherubism: Occurs in children; causes deformity but usually self limiting

Paget's Disease: In the elderly; commoner elsewhere in skeleton; often mild and asymptomatic

Non-Odontogenic Cysts with Epithelial Lining

Nasopalatine Duct Cyst: in the midline of the palate; may be mistaken for a periapical lucency and must be distinguished from normal nasopalatine duct.

Nasolabial Cyst: rare; seen in soft tissue in nasolabial fold.

Sublingual Dermoid: Presents as swelling in floor of mouth; arises deep beneath tongue; arises from pharyngeal arch; has thick lining and contains thick keratin

radiolucency in the midline of the palate and can easily be mistaken for a periapical lucency related to an incisor tooth or the normal naso-palatine duct. If more than 7 mm's diameter the lucency probably represents a cyst.

For the sake of being complete we mention the nasolabial cyst and sublingual dermoid which are cysts that neither present as radiolucencies nor as swellings of the jaws but as swelling adjacent to the jaws. They are rare and you are unlikely to see them.

Stafne's bone cavity, sometime called a cyst, is seen as a lucency in the posterior mandible and is not a cyst but a lucency caused by ectopic salivary tissue in the mandible. The appearance is usually enough to make a diagnosis and no further treatment is needed.

A traumatic bone cyst, also called a simple cyst, is also not a proper cyst (a pseudocyst). It is uncommon and seen in predominantly young people, usually seen in the anterior mandible around tooth roots without causing displacement or resorption of them. It is considered to be caused by some previous trauma. The lesion must be investigated surgically which reveals an empty bone cavity with no cyst lining or

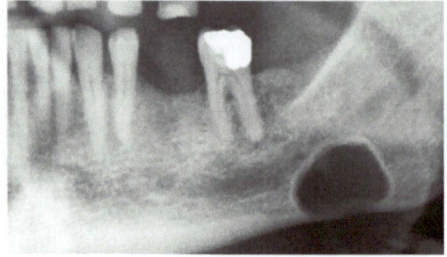
Stafne's bone cavity, not a cyst

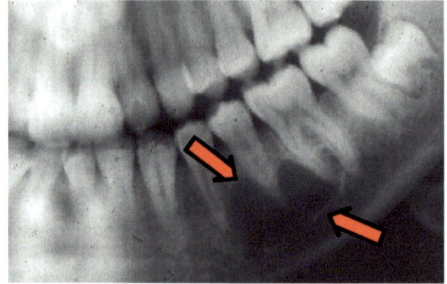
Traumatic or simple bone cyst, again not a real cyst

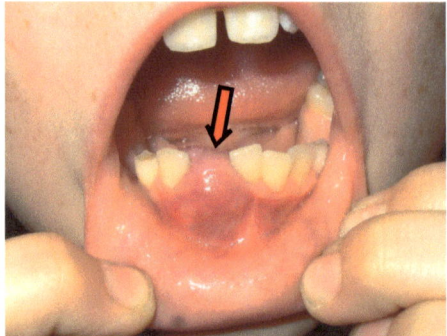
Central giant cell granuloma

fluid. The surgery will cause bleeding into the cavity which will reorganise into woven bone and eventually normality.

An aneurysmal bone cyst is a rare cause of painless swelling; curettage of the bloody cellular contents is usually curative.

When operating on any cystic lesion it should be aspirated with a needle and syringe as rarely a central jaw haematoma may be found. If the aspirate produces red arterial blood the procedure must be abandoned and the patient referred to an interventional radiologist for investigation and embolization before any further surgery.

Giant Cell Reparative Granuloma

We have previously mentioned the common peripheral giant cell granuloma arising as an epulis on the gingivae (chapter 18). The central giant cell granuloma occurs within the bone, most usually in the anterior mandible of a young person. It may present as a lucency on a radiograph or as a swelling. The treatment is surgical curettage. Histologically it is the same as the aforementioned epulis. There is a condition known as a 'brown tumour' associated with hyperparathyroidism which has the same histological appearance. This is very rare but in exams you should say that the patient's serum calcium should be tested to rule out hyperparathyroidism. In practice the patient will have presented and been diagnosed from other symptoms before this stage.

Cancer

We have previously mentioned osteo sarcoma affecting the jaws but this is quite rare; the mandible is more likely to be involved. The mandible and maxilla may be infiltrated with tumour in advanced intra-oral squamous cancer. Carcinoma of the maxillary antrum often presents as a painful swelling of the maxillary alveolus. Other distant cancers can metastasise to the jaws, particularly prostate, breast, kidney and thyroid. Usually there will be a radiolucency with an indistinct margin. The patient will probably have already had a diagnosis of one of these tumours, in which

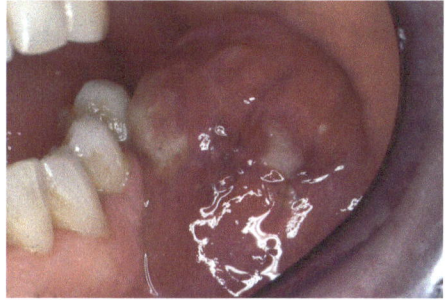

A metastatic adenocarcinoma from the gut

case they should be referred back to their oncologist. However this is not always the case; metastases can occur from occult primaries. A full history may reveal the site; a biopsy should be carried out with care as renal metastases can be very vascular and bleed a lot. Numbness of the infra-orbital or mental nerve suggests a sinister diagnosis.

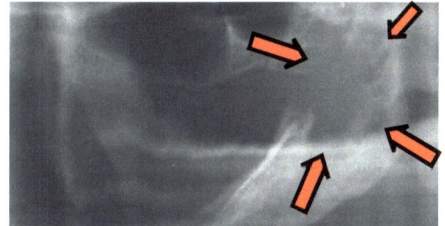

Prostatic carcinoma metastasis in left mandibular ramus. The patient reported a loud crack from his jaw when eating as his mandible fractured. The red arrows indicate the indistinct margins of the cancer

Paget's disease

Described by Sir James Paget in the 1870s as 'osteitis deformans' the disease causes abnormality of bone remodelling with dysfunctional resorption and new bone apposition. It leads to bone swelling, pain and deformity. Only the elderly are affected and, although it is not uncommon and it can affect the jaws, most cases are asymptomatic and may be seen on X-rays taken for other purposes but generally infrequently in the jaws. In the unlikely event that a patient presents with it in the jaws extractions are likely to be problematical as the bone will be brittle and fragile.

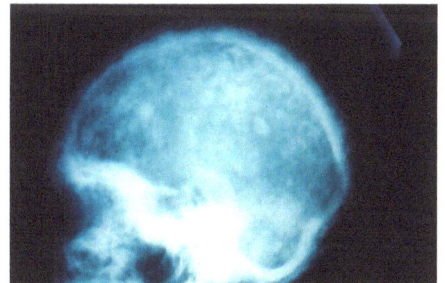

A very marked case of Paget's in the skull. The patient had a significantly swollen maxilla. Diagnosis was confirmed by a very raised serum alkaline phosphatase level which indicates marked bone resorption and deposition

22 Salivary Gland Swelling

The commonest salivary swellings are mucous extravasation and retention cysts. The remainder will mostly be related to inflammation or neoplasia. You should be able to recognise a mucous cyst and distinguish it from an infective swelling and a neoplastic one. A mucous cyst will usually be in the lip or floor of mouth, be soft, have a bluish tinge and obviously contain fluid. An infective swelling will usually have a short history and be tender or painful, and a neoplastic one will be slow growing and non-tender; pain will occur in malignant disease but only when the lesion is more advanced.

Mucosal Cysts

Mucosal cysts are commonly found in the lip. The most common is the mucous extravasation cyst which occurs when the small ducts from the mucous glands in the lower lip become damaged by trauma from the teeth and the mucus is discharged into the soft tissue of the lip causing an unsightly blue swelling which itself will become traumatised. A mucous retention cyst is where the duct is damaged and the mucus accumulates in the gland which itself swells. The distinction is only made histologically.

Any attempt to puncture the cyst to release the mucus will be followed by recurrence. Surgery should be carried out to remove the small mucous gland which is feeding the cyst. This is not straightforward as there are many dozens of them and it is important to get the right one. A vertical incision should be used, followed by blunt dissection to avoid damage to the small vertical nerves that supply sensation to the vermillion of the lip which can easily be damaged in this procedure.

A ranula is a retention cyst of the sublingual salivary gland; again treatment is by removing the gland. The sublingual gland does not shell out easily; it requires

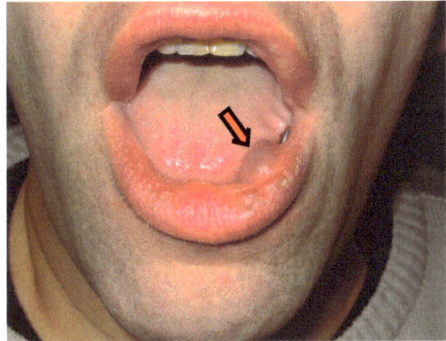

Mucous cyst

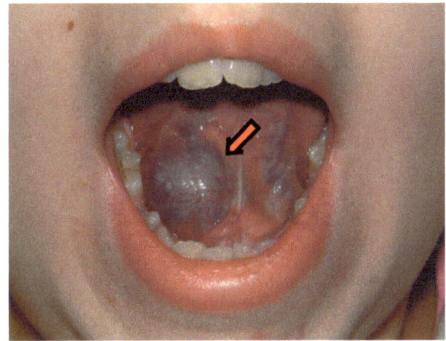

Ranula

more of a controlled tearing which may lead to bleeding so general anaesthetic is preferred. A plunging ranula is where the cyst penetrates the mylohyoid muscle and presents as a soft cyst in the neck. Treatment is the same: removal of the sublingual gland from within the mouth.

Inflammatory Salivary Gland Swelling

This may be due to viral infection, most especially mumps in children, but now of very low incidence due to MMR vaccination. More commonly it will be due to bacterial infection. This may occur when there is a low salivary flow rate such as if the patient is dehydrated, particularly if they are acutely ill or immunocompromised. However the majority of cases of acutely infected glands will be related to salivary obstruction which becomes secondarily infected; this is more common in the submandibular glands

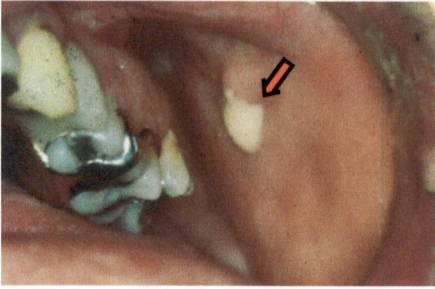

Pus discharging from the parotid duct which opens opposite the first molar tooth

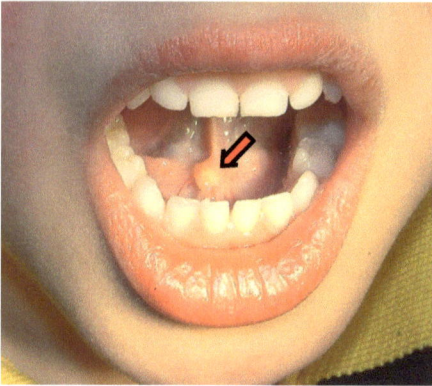

A calculus lodged at the punctum of the submandibular duct. This was easily removed using local anaesthetic and the obstruction relieved

where calculi are most common, although they can occur also in the parotid glands where there can also be obstruction caused by strictures in the duct.

Patients commonly present with submandibular swelling related to eating which is usually caused by obstruction from a calculus, sometimes in the deep part of the gland but more usually in the duct in the floor of the mouth. An X-ray may show the stone, but this is not reliable as it may not be opaque enough to show, but it may often be palpable or even visible at the punctum of the duct. This is sometimes referred to as 'meal time syndrome'; it frequently leads to secondary infection so that the symptoms are caused by obstruction and inflammation from infection.

Occasionally a patient may have recurrent sialadentis which may require

---

Commonest Salivary Swellings

Cyst:

Mucous extravasation or retention cyst: Usually in the lower lip

Ranula: Mucous cyst of sublingual gland

Infective:

Submandibular sialadentitis: Usually secondary to obstruction from a calculus

Parotid sialadenitis: Secondary to obstruction from duct stricture or calculus

(Sialadentitis related to viral infection, dehydration or acute illness is much less common and unlikely to be seen in dental practice)

Benign tumours:

Pleomorphic salivary adenoma: most common and usually in parotid; can turn malignant; can recur if not removed with a good margin

Warthin's tumour: most common in parotid

Malignant:

Squamous carcinoma from pleomorphic adenoma: most common in parotid

Muco-epidermoid carcinoma: three grades of malignancy: low grade (fairly benign), intermediate and high grade behaving like squamous cell carcinoma

Adenocystic carcinoma: Invades slowly particularly along nerves; very high 5 year survival but recurs many years later

----

There are a large number of rarer salivary tumours

---

gland removal. Recurrent sialadentis in children can occur but is very rare and usually self-limiting as they grow.

Salivary tumours

These are most commonly benign and most frequent in the parotid gland. There are a variety of benign salivary tumours but the pleomorphic adenoma is the commonest, followed by the Warthin's tumour. Pleomorphic adenomas, although benign, tend to propagate cells beyond their apparent capsule so that they can easily recur and they can also turn into malignant squamous carcinomas. Warthin's tumours are the next most common, also benign. It is not essential to remove them but if they are visible on the face they may be removed for cosmesis. Warthin's can be bilateral and can sometimes cause pain which would be an indication for removal; they most frequently affect women and are associated with smoking.

Tumours in the sublingual and submandibular glands are less common but are more likely to be malignant. Following squamous carcinoma arising from pleomorphic adenomas the most common malignant tumours are the mucoepidermoid tumour and the adenocystic carcinoma. Mucoepidermoid tumours have different grades of malignancy. Some low grade tumours behave as almost benign; intermediate grade tumours are truly malignant and behave like squamous cell carcinomas and high grade are very nasty. Adenocystic carcinomas spread very slowly along nerves. Once adequately removed their 5 year survival rate is nearly 100% but they tend to recur many years later at distant sites having invaded along nerves.

As we have already seen in chapter 18 tumours can all occur in the minor salivary glands particularly in the palate.

Examination

You should enquire about the duration of symptoms, the presence and nature of any pain and you should palpate the parotid and submandibular glands. When examining the submandibular glands you should palpate bimanually with a gloved finger in the floor of the mouth and another

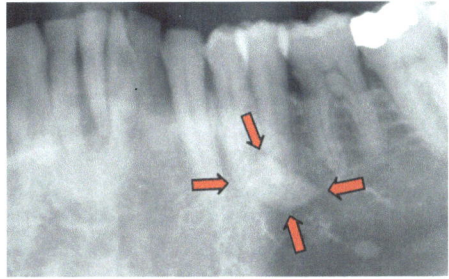

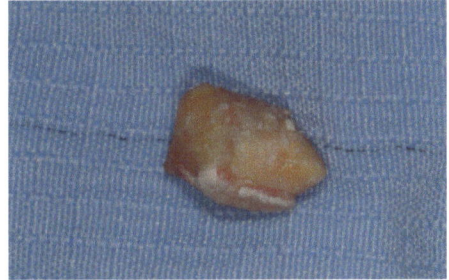

Submandibular calculi can be radiopaque as this one seen in the detail from a panoral X-ray (top). Below: the calculus after removal from the floor of the mouth

in the submandibular area. You are looking to elicit the degree of any swelling comparing the two sides, the consistency of any swelling and tenderness. You should look out for any hard lumps in the floor of the mouth anteriorly, which might suggest a calculus in the submandibular duct, or posteriorly in the floor of mouth which might indicate a stone in the deep part of the submandibular gland. Occasionally a calculus may lodge in the papilla of the parotid duct.

Examination of the parotid gland should include an assessment for mouth opening and facial nerve weakness (a malignant tumour can compromise the facial nerve which passes through the gland) and an examination of the soft palate. A tumour in the deep part of the parotid gland can press on the soft palate and present as a swelling there. The whole palate should be examined for tumours in the minor salivary glands.

Management

Salivary tumours may be investigated with computerised tomography or magnetic resonance imaging. However imaging for swellings is primarily by ultrasound. This will tell the clinician whether the swelling is multifocal, bilateral, the size and whether it originates in the salivary tissue or in the lymph glands within the parotid gland which may be enlarged by metastatic squamous cancer from the skin.

Fine needle aspiration cytology is usually used to elicit the type of tumour; this can be guided using ultrasound.

Tumours should be surgically removed. Pleomorphic adenomas, the commonest, should be removed with a good margin of normal tissue to prevent recurrence. In practice this will mean a superficial parotidectomy if in the parotid gland, the most common site. Most tumours are in the superficial 5/6th of the gland which is that part superficial to the facial nerve which passes through it. If the tumour involves the deep part of the gland it should all be removed which carries a risk of facial nerve damage. Surgery for removal of the sublingual, submandibular or minor salivary glands is less problematic. Pleomorphic adenomas should be removed promptly after diagnosis as they can develop squamous cell carcinomas within them.

In the most common case of obstruction which occurs in the submandibular gland a calculus can often be felt in the floor of the mouth. Sometimes it may be visible on a plain X-ray but not necessarily. Sometimes it can be retrieved through an incision in the floor of the mouth which relieves the obstruction and symptoms. The patient should be warned that further stones may form later. A calculus may be visualised through a sialoscope and retrieved with a small basket. Sometimes it is necessary to remove the gland because of recurrent stones or sialadentis.

Obstruction of the outflow of the parotid gland may be due to a stricture more commonly than a stone. This may be demonstrated with sialography where a

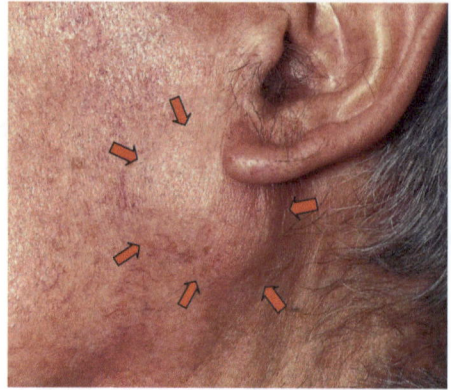

A tumour in the tail of the parotid gland presenting as a slowly enlarging painless swelling. This was a pleomorphic adenoma. Parotid swellings may arise from lymph nodes within the gland and be caused by lymphomas or metastatic skin cancer from around the ear

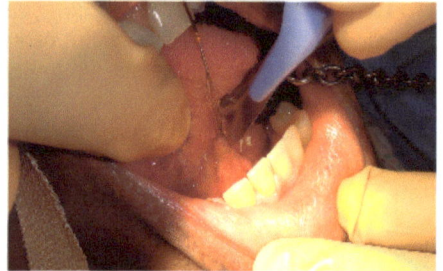

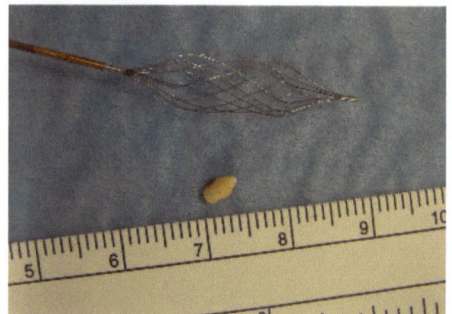

Basket retrieval of a submandibular stone. The punctum of the duct is incised to allow the basket to be fed into the duct (top). Below: the basket and retrieved calculus

radiopaque contrast is injected into the duct to enable an image of the ductal system to be made with X-rays. This may be therapeutic as well as diagnostic as it may flush out plugs of mucus which are causing obstruction. Strictures can often be treated by dilatation with a fine catheter or injection of saline into the duct and irrigation with a little pressure.

23 Jaw Fractures

Fractures of the jaws usually present to hospital departments of emergency medicine but sometimes they may present to a dental surgery when the patient is aware of a dental injury but not that their jaw is broken.

Most jaw fractures occur as a result of interpersonal violence, falls and sporting injuries, but some still occur as a result of road traffic accidents, though significantly less than in the days before cars had seat belts, air bags and crumple zones.

Mandibular Fractures

Fractures of the mandible are quite common. The lower jaw usually breaks at its weakest point which is the neck of the mandibular condyle. The patient will have discomfort and swelling around the jaw and pain on opening the mouth as limitation of mouth opening and lateral jaw movement. Typically the dental occlusion will be deranged and on attempting to open the jaw will move towards the affected side.

Diagnosis of a fracture is usually confirmed by an orthopantomograph X-ray. A simple undisplaced fracture may be managed conservatively with the patient having a soft diet and analgesia for a few days. Where there is derangement of the occlusion the fracture may be managed with intermaxillary fixation with wires but where the fragments are severely displaced, particularly with the ends overriding or there are bilateral fractures, then open reduction and fixation with miniplates is the usual treatment.

After the condyle fractures at the angle of the mandible are the next commonest because the mandible is often weakened at this position by unerupted third molar teeth. Again the patient will have discomfort and swelling and probably derangement of the occlusion. Sometimes the fracture may be a simple crack and undisplaced with no occlusal derangement, in which case it may be managed conservatively with a soft diet

Jaw Fractures Symptoms & Signs
• Extra-oral swelling or lacerations
• Tenderness on palpation
• Limitation mouth opening or lateral movement
• Dysaesthesia of mental nerve (angle and body fracture)
• Dental injury
• Intra-oral swelling or bruising
• Mobile teeth
• Gingival lacerations
• Occlusal derangement
• Movement between fragments

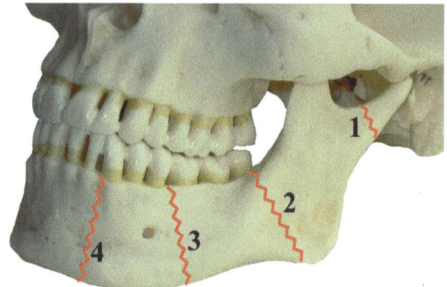

Mandibular fractures: 1. Condyle 2: Angle 3: Body 4: Paraymphyseal

only. In this circumstance it is usual for the patient to be prescribed antibiotics with analgesics as all mandibular fractures other than condylar are compound into the mouth and the presence of unerupted teeth will facilitate infection. Body and parasymphyseal fractures are the most likely to present at a dental surgery as the patient may be aware of a loose tooth but be unaware that this is because of a break.

Patients suspected of having a fracture should be examined for swelling intra and extra-orally, limitation of mouth opening and lateral movement, lacerations within and outside the mouth, bleeding into the mouth and most particularly derangement of the occlusion. Angle and body fractures

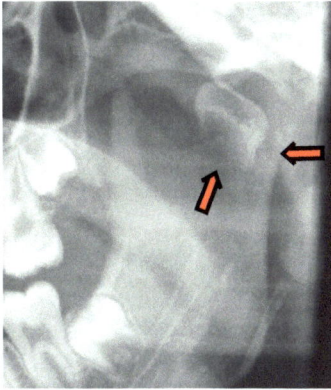
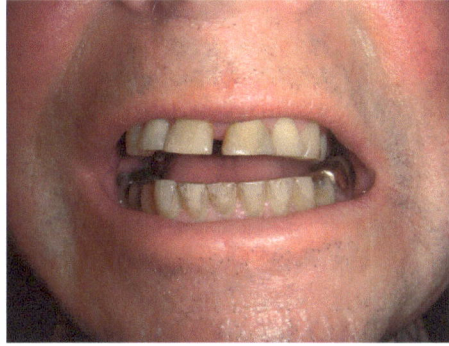

Fracture of the left mandibular condyle causing shortening of the left mandibular ramus seen on X-ray and clinically as premature occlusal contact on the left hand side

may be accompanied by dysaesthesia of the mental nerve as the nerve may be stretched in the inferior dental canal if the fracture is displaced.

The aim of treatment is primarily to restore the dental occlusion as even small discrepancies may be uncomfortable for the patient. This is normally achieved by reduction of the fracture and fixation with titanium miniplates. Lacerations are closed with sutures, and teeth which are damaged beyond repair are removed. If the patient is treated soon after injury then teeth in the line of the fracture need not necessarily be removed if they will continue to be functional. If treatment is delayed then they may facilitate infection and may best be extracted.

It is optimal for fractures of the mandible to be treated within 24 hours of injury. But unless there is severe displacement of the fragments or there are loose teeth that might obstruct the patient's airways or be inhaled then they are not considered to be medical emergencies.

Before titanium miniplates became available it was usual for fractures to be fixed with intermaxillary fixation with wires, splints or arch bars wired to the teeth. These methods have fallen into disuse now but it is still possible to manage most simple jaw fractures with

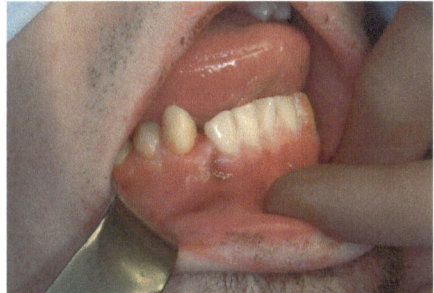
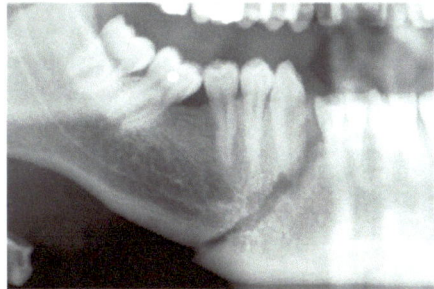
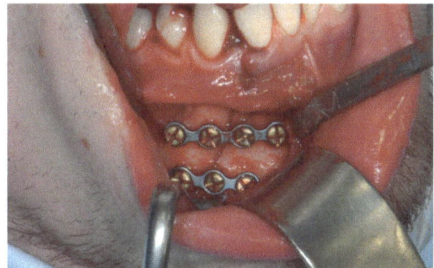

Parasymphyseal fracture of mandible. Occlusal derangement and gingival laceration (top), Detail of panoral image (middle), titanium miniplates in position at operation before closing (bottom)

intermaxillary fixation with 'eyelet' wires using local anaesthetic in a dental surgery without hospital admission. This method has the advantage of being easy, quick, cheap and with minimised delay.

Fractures of the Maxilla

Fractures of the maxilla are much less common than those of the mandible, partly because the midface (excepting the zygoma) is less exposed to a fist or in a fall and partly because a great force is required to injure it. Maxillary fractures have traditionally been classified as Le Fort 1, 2 or 3. However in practice there is usually some comminution of the bone fragments and it is possible for fractures to occur at more than one of these levels on the same side and at different levels on opposite sides. Le Fort 1 fracture is uncommon because it requires a concentrated severe force just above the roots of the teeth; Le Fort 2 is the least uncommon and Le Fort 3 is a complete separation of the mid-face from the cranial base and is a severe injury.

Maxillary fractures are more likely to need emergency management than mandibles as the airway may be obstructed and because they are more likely to be accompanied by other injuries. They may particularly be associated with head injuries. These may produce an intracranial haemorrhage giving neurological signs and needing a CT scan to assess the injury or they may be more subtle leading to no obvious neurological deficit but to a small change in personality or decrease in intellectual capacity afterwards.

A maxillary fracture is easily diagnosed by examination. The examiner should steady the nasal bridge with one gloved hand to see if there is a differential movement of the maxilla with the other hand. Of course there may be dental injuries and derangement of the occlusion. There will be bleeding into the nasal cavity but this is usually not severe; if it should be so the nose can be packed to aid haemostasis. Further assessment is by CT scan; it is most

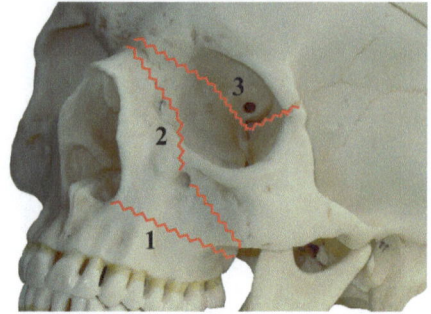

Maxillary fractures: Le Fort 1, 2 & 3

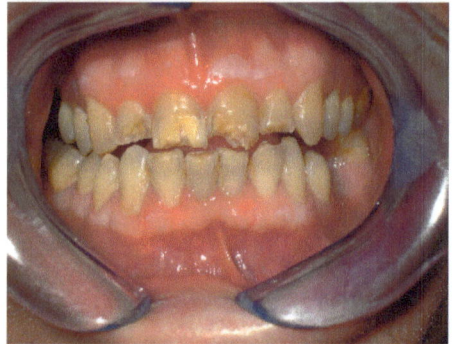

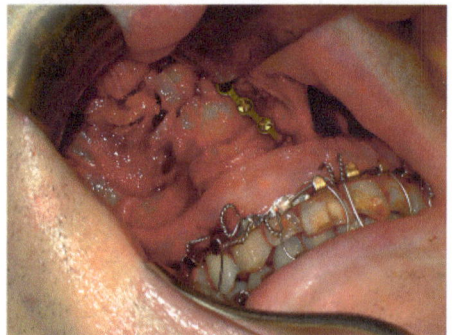

A maxillary fracture two weeks after injury. The incisors are damaged and the occlusion is altered but it has been partly reduced by biting forces leaving an anterior open bite (above). At operation the fracture has been reduced by applying intermaxillary fixation with arch bars and wires. Miniplates have been used to secure the fragments; the intermaxillary fixation can then be removed at the end of the operation

useful when the image is reconstituted into 3 dimensions to plan treatment.

Once it is clear that the airway is safe the definitive treatment can be delayed without disadvantage until after other possibly life endangering injuries have been dealt with. Treatment is usually fixation of the fractures with titanium miniplates.

Dento-alveolar Fractures

Fractures of the teeth with displacement and fracture of the alveolar bone but without a complete break through the mandible are most commonly in the anterior of the mouth They should be treated swiftly, usually in the dental surgery, by repositioning the teeth and fractured bone into position. The fractured teeth and segment of bone can then be fixed with a splint or more commonly with wire fixed between the teeth or attached by an acid etch technique as below. These fractures should be treated as soon as possible after injury to reduce the chance of teeth becoming non vital or infected.

Dental Trauma

Teeth that have been traumatised should be assessed and managed immediately to give the best long term prognosis. The principal complications to avoid, if possible, are loss of vitality and root resorption.

Where the crowns have been fractured and dentine exposed the teeth should be dressed and if the pulps are exposed they will need to be extirpated and the root canal dressed or filled. If the alveolus is fractured and displaced it should be repositioned and splinted, usually with wire to the adjacent teeth.

Teeth that have been displaced (luxated) should be reduced into their correct position and splinted to adjacent teeth. This is best achieved with stainless steel orthodontic wire attached by acid etch composite for a period of 4 weeks. The aim is to secure the teeth but not so rigidly that there is no physiological movement of the tooth within the periodontal ligament. A rigidly splinted tooth has a higher risk of becoming ankylosed in the bone and of resorbing later.

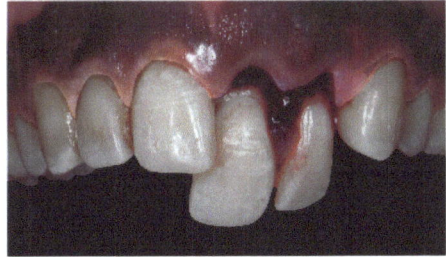

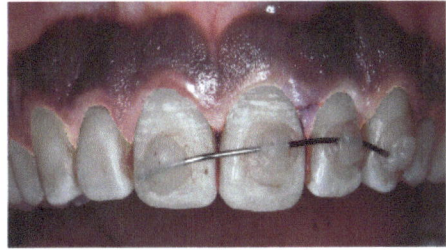

Severely displaced (luxated) teeth repositioned and splinted with orthodontic wire attached with acid etched composite See the technique at: https://vimeo.com/137957560

Teeth that have been traumatised but not displaced (concussed) need no active splinting and where the tooth is loosened but not displaced (subluxed) splinting may be placed for two weeks to decrease discomfort in function. Traumatised teeth will need to be followed up with periodic vitality testing and radiographic examination to check for root resorption.

Teeth that have been completely avulsed can be washed gently with water or saline, without touching the root, reimplanted and splinted with a flexible splint for between one and two weeks. Reimplantation will be more successful with teeth with an open apex in younger patients.

Examination tips:

• Know the aetiology and clinical features of mandibular fractures

• Be familiar with the types of dental trauma and how to manage them in a timely fashion

• The management of dental trauma may be examined in 'restorative' examinations

24 Biopsy

Tissue is frequently removed from the mouth for examination by a histopathologist in both oral medicine and oral surgery practice. Apart from fine needle aspiration cytology the techniques are easy to master and will be described here. We submit almost all tissue removed during surgery for pathological examination, with the exception of extracted teeth. The purpose is to help with a diagnosis where this is otherwise uncertain or unknown, to confirm a diagnosis we are already fairly certain of but wish to confirm and to check the margins of excision which is most important in managing malignant disease.

Histopathology reports come with a description of the tissues examined, both the macroscopic appearance of the specimen before it has been processed and the cellular appearance after the specimen has been fixed, embedded in wax blocks and cut into sections to be viewed under the microscope. The pathologist's diagnosis must be considered with the clinical history and features in making a final working diagnosis. The histopathology may be inaccurate, particularly if the specimen is too small, taken from an unrepresentative area of the lesion or in the presence of acute inflammation. Requests must be accompanied with a brief clinical history for the pathologist to interpret the microscopic findings.

There are four techniques in frequent use. Incision biopsy is where a specimen is from part of a lesion. Usually a wedge is taken which includes a representative part of the lesion, its margin and some normal tissue from the edge. A wedge shape facilitates closure with sutures. Excision biopsy is used when there is a clinically benign lesion; the intention is to remove the lesion whole as the definitive treatment and the specimen is examined to confirm a diagnosis. A punch biopsy is taken with a

Information needed with a histopathology request:
- Patient's demographic details
- Specimen and request clearly labelled
- Brief description of lesion
- Brief history of complaint
- Smoking, drinking & medication where relevant
- Results of other investigations
- Provisional clinical diagnosis

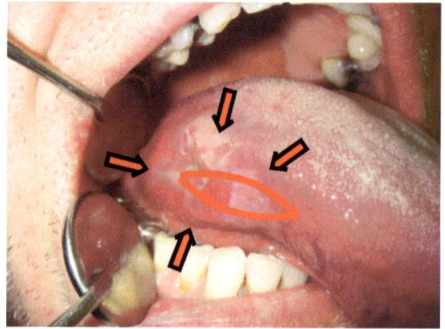

Incision margins for incision biopsy of this obvious squamous cancer of the lateral margin of the tongue. The macroscopic margins of the tumour are marked with arrows

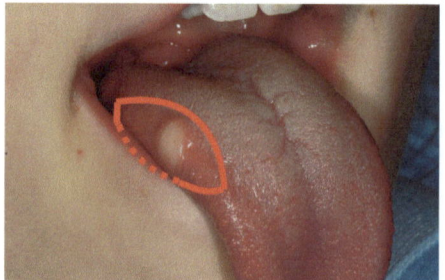

This lesion has all the clinical features of being benign so it is going to be removed completely. The incision margins for this excision biopsy are marked

3 mm diameter punch (usually) or a 5 mm and is particularly useful for lesions of the attached gingiva or where we want multiple samples from different parts of a lesion such as large areas of potentially dysplastic epithelium. <u>Fine needle aspiration cytology</u> is used for suspected salivary swellings or enlarged lymph nodes in the neck. This requires additional experience to get a representative sample; it can be performed using ultrasound to accurately target the needle.

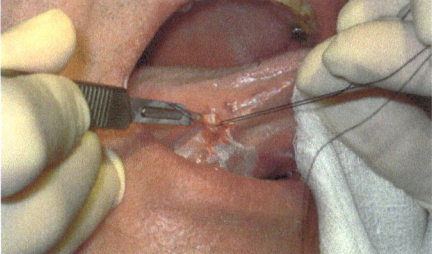

Any suspicious lesion should have a biopsy specimen taken for examination with a microscope. Here an incisional biopsy is is being taken. Part of the lesion, a floor of mouth keratosis, is being removed from the margin with some normal tissue

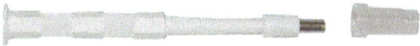

A 3mm biopsy punch

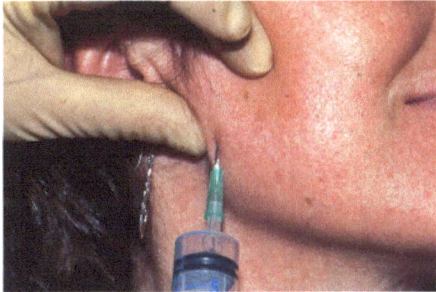

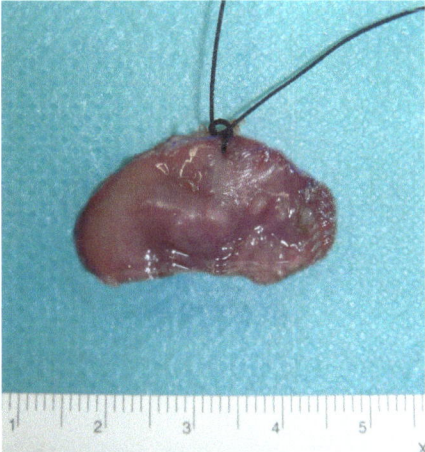

This specimen has been marked with a suture so the pathologist can orientate which way round it is

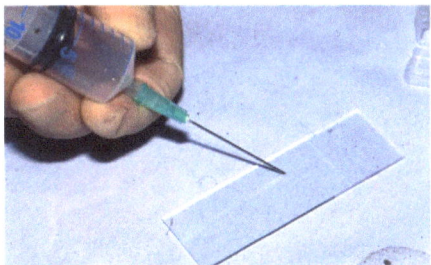

Fine needle aspiration cytology. A sample is taken from a parotid tumour (above) and gently put onto a slide to go to the laboratory

Appendix 1 Assessment

During your undergraduate course you will be subjected to a number of different assessments designed to help you and to help your teachers to help you progress to the required standard, to ensure that you have learned the skills necessary to participate in patient treatment and finally to assess whether you are safe to practise as a newly qualified dental surgeon.

Clinical ability tests

These are in course assessments which involve set tasks to perform under supervision during a time of your own choosing in the clinic. They may involve such matters as: giving a local anaesthetic, disposing of sharps safely, preparing a patient for surgery, understanding the procedures for cross infection control, choosing which instruments to use, obtaining consent and giving post-operative instructions. You will carry out a task while being observed by a tutor and being asked some questions concerning essential background knowledge. You should expect to be marked and be given feedback on areas in which you may be able to improve. These skills will all be on subjects that will become second nature after a while and which you will come to carry out efficiently without conscious thought.

Example: clinical ability test

Title: Clinical Ability Test - Minor Oral Surgery

Aim: Appraisal of student's ability to surgically remove a tooth or root

Test: Assess ability to - take a history and present the case, consent the patients for the procedure, carry out a surgical procedure to remove a tooth or root under local anaesthetic, deliver appropriate post-operative care, and test the knowledge of suture materials and techniques.

Marks are awarded for:

Introduction of patient: patient's name, age & occupation

Confirmation of: referral source, complaint, relevant medical history, diagnosis & treatment plan.

Justification of treatment plan: indications for removal of the tooth, alternative treatment plans

Consent: with appropriate warnings of sequelae/complications

Compliance with cross infection guidelines

Good organisation of the surgical site and instruments

Extraction of tooth competently: raise appropriately designed flap, use of drill to remove appropriate amount of bone, correct choice of elevators/forceps, correct use of instruments with appropriate measures taken to minimize trauma to local tissues, delivery of tooth with good control and suitable force, wound toilet, suture flap - knowledge of suture materials and indications for use of each, check for haemostasis.

Administer post operative instructions.

Written: Short answer questions

Written papers are unlikely to require an answer in essay format. Short answer questions are usually used in which a clinical scenario is described followed by short concise questions which should be answered in a paragraph and for which marks are awarded according to criteria set in advance for the examiner who is marking. There will be a series of such questions, most usually 20 all of which must be answered. Marks are awarded on defined criteria that have been agreed by a committee of examiners beforehand so that a standard has been defined for the pass mark.

Example: minor oral surgery short answer question

You plan to extract the unrestorable lower right second premolar of a fit and healthy 23 year old man in your dental surgery. His remaining dentition is unrestored and there is no other dental disease evident either clinically or radiographically.

1. List 4 possible factors that you may have elicited from this patient's history and examination which would indicate this premolar extraction would require minor oral surgery. (2 marks)

2. Give 2 indications for raising a mucoperiosteal flap after the crown fractures whilst you're attempting to extract the lower second premolar. (2 marks)

3. Draw a diagram of the surgical site and indicate on it the positions of the incisions that you would make to raise a mucoperiosteal flap. Explain your reasoning for the positioning of the incisions. (8 marks)

4. Following removal of the tooth you wish to close the wound. Which type of suture would you select to do this? Please include the material, needle shape and body design and gauge of suture that you would select. (2 marks)

5. What analgesic regime would you recommend for this patient? Please include drug name, dose, frequency, route and duration. (4 marks)

6. Give 4 other indications (other than surgical removal of a tooth) for raising a flap in this region. (2 marks)

Single best answer multiple choice

Multiple choice questions are usually marked by a computer and usually of the single best answer variety. There will be a stem to the question in the form of a short clinical vignette of one or two sentences with 5 possible responses, only one of which is correct. A mark is awarded for choosing the correct answer; there is no negative mark for a wrong answer and no marks are awarded if more than one answer is chosen.

Example: single best answer multiple choice question

A patient who is taking warfarin with an INR of 3 attends for extraction of a lower right first molar tooth. Which actions would you take?

a. Pack with oxidised cellulose gauze and suture

b. Use Diathermy

c. Apply bone wax to socket

d. Give a vitamin K supplement

e. Reduce warfarin dose 2 day pre-op

Objective Structured Clinical Examination (OSCE)

These are clinically based tasks and usually involve one examiner observing each candidate perform each one. There is often a patient involved who is usually a paid professional actor. Marks are awarded according to pre-set defined criteria and if there is a patient (actor) there are always soft marks for introducing yourself nicely, explaining what you are proposing to do. Normally there will be a series of these and the candidates will rotate from one 'station' to another usually at 10 minute intervals.

Candidates are normally given one or two minutes to read an instruction sheet before entering the 'station'. There will be about 6 minutes for the task and a couple for change over to the next station.

OSCE stations require some considerable preparation on the part of the examiners and support staff to set them up, and not inconsiderable imagination to think up new tasks that are going to be of value. You can therefore expect a lot of repetition of stations between different exams. There is usually one on washing hands correctly, resuscitating a manikin, consenting a patient for a procedure, counselling a patient with a complication. Always read the task carefully and do what you are requested. If the question tells you to take a history you will be awarded marks for the various stages of history taking; you will probably get a mark for discovering something important or relevant but the marking will be on the process of taking the history.

Example: OSCE station

Aim: To test competency of candidate to demonstrate communication with patients and knowledge of effects of bisphosphate on jaws and implications for dental treatment

Scenario (Candidate's instructions): A 63 year old lady with a history of toothache from a lower molar presents to your surgery requesting an extraction. She gives a history of breast cancer with metastatic disease for which she has monthly infusion of zoledronic acid (Zometa). An panoral radiograph is provided. Take a medical history and discuss the options for treatment.

List of Equipment: paper, pencil, chair, table, panoral radiograph, actor to play role of patient

Actor's Instructions: Judith Green aged 63 <u>Occupation</u>- Housekeeper works in hospital for last 15 years <u>Presenting History</u>- You have had pain in the lower molar tooth on and off for several weeks; initially the tooth was sensitive to hot and cold then became painful to bite on and now there is a constant dull pain. <u>Past Medical History</u> 2 years ago had pain in leg; bone cancer was diagnosed; has monthly infusions through a drip at the hospital. Now OK no pain.

<u>Medication:</u> Zoledronic acid Zometa (Bisphosphonates) infusion once each month for the bone cancer.

Marks awarded for: Candidate introduces him / herself to patient.

Candidate invites questions and encourages discourse, faces 'patient' and makes eye contact; candidate uses appropriate language for a lay person, explains the problem, explains the treatment options

Candidate gives an understandable explanation of problem, discussion & plan for immediate pain relief, extirpates pulp to relieve pain, explains the problem of medication, advises patient of risk of bone necrosis, discussion about tooth extraction, extraction of tooth is contraindicated because of risk of bone necrosis

Extended Matching Questions

These are multiple choice questions which can test details of knowledge. They are organised into sets that use the same list of options. The number of questions and options can vary from one set to the next with anything from 2 to 10 questions for each option set. The questions will have a theme, candidate instructions, a list of options, and at least two scenarios.

Example: extended matching question

Theme: Investigations before minor oral surgery

Lead-in statement: For each patient requiring minor oral surgery, select the most appropriate investigation from the option list. Each option might be used once, more than once, or not at all.

Option list:

A)   Full blood count

b)   Panoral radiograph

c)   INR

d)   Blood electrolytes

e)   Cone beam CT scan

f)   Periapical radiograph

g)   Hepatitis B serology

h)   Blood glucose

i)   Coagulation screen

Scenarios:

1. *A 57 woman with a painful loose lower 6*

2. *A 24 year old healthy woman with an impacted third molar*

3. *An elderly gentleman presenting with a swollen face and trismus*

4. *A 73 year old man needing a dental clearance*

5. *A healthy patient presenting with continuous severe bleeding after an extraction*

6. *A patient on warfarin who needs a lower premolar removed*

Clinical cases

These may be 'seen' cases where the candidates present patients in their final examinations that they have treated usually in restorative dentistry. They will normally be asked questions by the examiners and have to discuss what they have done and then justify the treatment plan and possible alternatives.

They may also be presented with 'unseen' cases where they are presented with a patient they have not met before and are observed by the examiners as they take a history and examine them in a dental chair prescribed as in written instructions they have seen before. They are marked as they go along a variety of different domains, such as communication, clinical knowledge etc.

Viva Voce

Viva examinations usually involve a candidate being asked questions by two examiners. The candidate may be described a clinical scenario, sometimes with photographs, study models or radiographs. This is usually highly structured with the examiners asking questions from a prepared list and marking according to a concise scheme decided in advance. The two examiners usually mark independently and marks are pooled to produce an overall result. It is usual for individual examiners' marks to be looked at independently and if the examiner is an 'outlier' in the range of marks awarded their mark may be discarded as may marks for individual questions if a large number of candidates fail as it may indicate a question which is not assessing their knowledge and ability adequately.

Appendix 2 Dental Panoramic Tomograph Interpretation

Also called a 'panoral' or orthopantomograph (OPG), will provide a wealth of radiological information about pathology in the teeth and jaws and is the chief investigation used in oral surgery practice. However before requesting an X-ray dentists will need to consider the justification for it and record this in the patient's records. For X-ray to be justified the diagnostic benefit must outweigh the potential detriment of the radiation dose. All dentists (and students) should be aware of and follow the guidance in the Ionising Radiation (Medical Exposure) Regulations IR(ME)R. All radiation techniques used must use the lowest reasonable dose.

Thus intra oral periapical images should be used preferentially for images of single teeth if needed for diagnosis before extraction, if an X-ray is needed at all. Where more information is needed concerning the general oral condition then the increased X-ray dose of a panoral will be justified. If more than four periapical images are needed then a panoral will cause a lower dose of radiation.

Cone beam computerised tomography is becoming more commonly used in oral surgery practice. It can used for implant planning, localisation of canines and other impacted teeth and roots in the maxillary antrum. It can be used for assessment of medication related jaw necrosis and other bone pathology. However the radiation dose is often much greater than a panoral but depends on the equipment used.

The panoral is a tomogram, the principle of which is that the X-ray source and sensor rotate around the subject so that radiopaque structures (cervical spine in this case) not of interest are outside the focal trough. This decreases interference with the image of the area being examined.

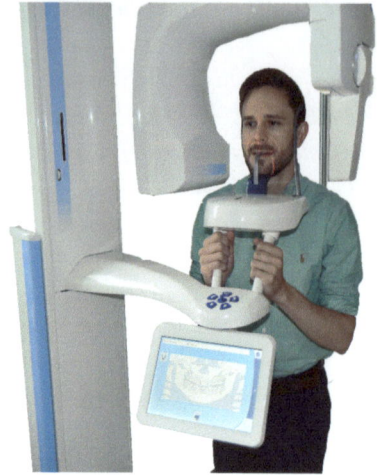

The patient is positioned in the panoral machine. The X-ray source and sensor rotate around the patient and give a clear image within a 'focal trough' containing the dentition and alveolar bone. Structures we have no interest in, particularly the cervical spine, are out of focus. However it still leaves the image in the centre less distinct than buccal structures

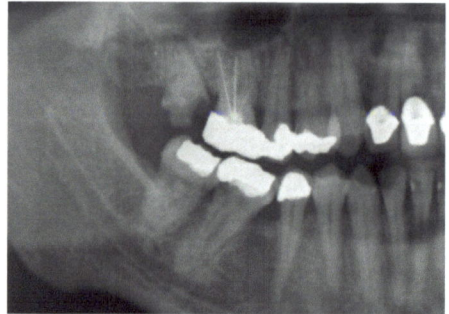

A modern digital panoral machine will give a very good image of dental disease such as the lucency above the upper 5 & 8 and caries beneath the lower 7 in a detail from the following image

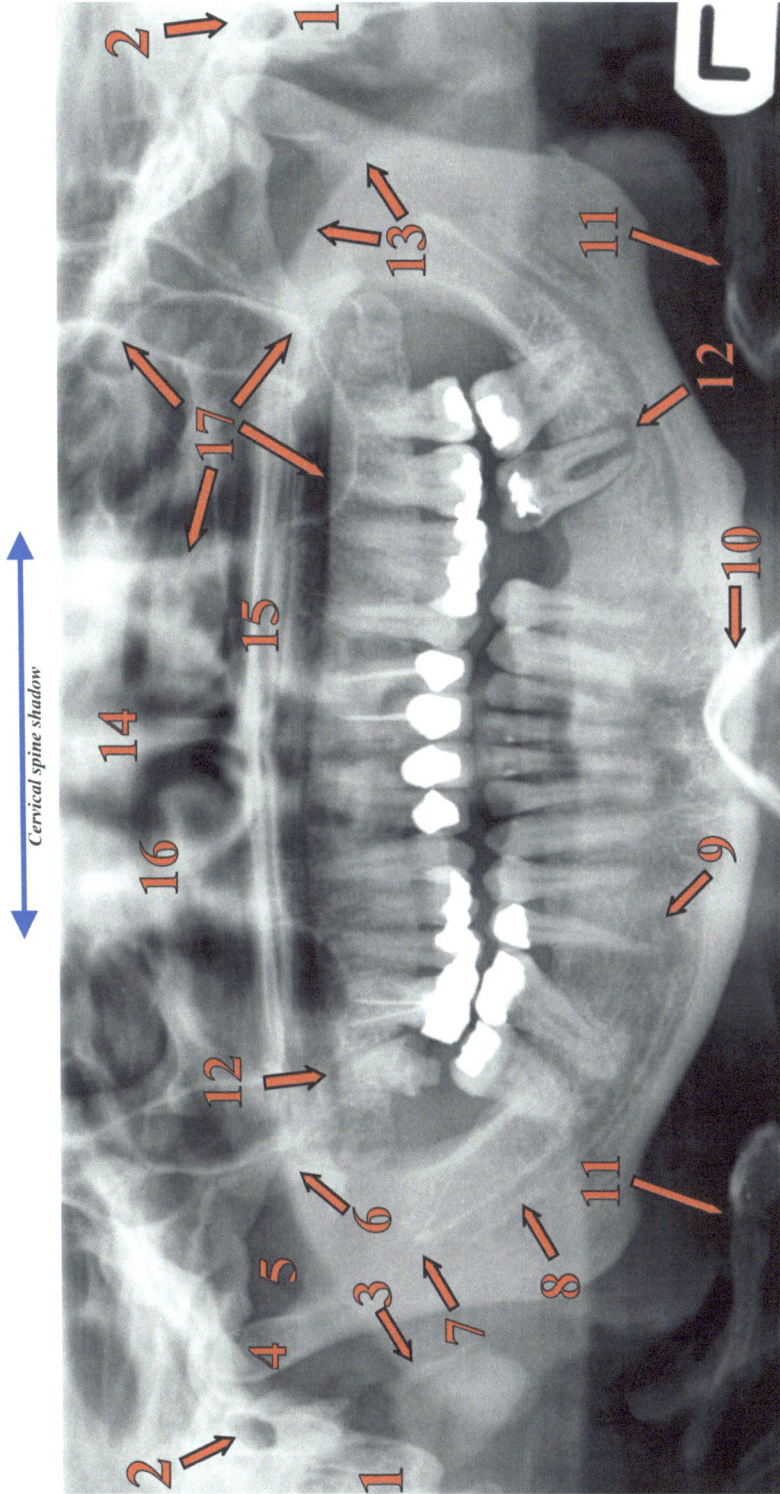

1: cervical spine 2: external auditory meatus 3: styloid process 4: mandibular condyle 5: sigmoid notch 6: coronoid process 7: lingula of mandible 8: inferior dental canal 9: mental foramen 10: artifact (necklace) 11: hyoid bone 12: apical lucency from non-vital tooth 13: pharyngeal air shadow 14: nasal septum 15: floor of nose 16: lateral margin nasal cavity/medial of antrum 17: maxillary antrum

Appendix 3 Guidance and Protocols

There are numerous guidelines and protocols available for medical and dental professionals and these are invaluable in giving guidance to best practice. They are usually drawn up by committees of specialists in the fields being examined and take into account recent research and advances. Their existence makes life much easier for the clinician as by following the guidance they can ensure they are providing current approved treatment without having to be up to date with all the latest research papers and primary evidence themselves. Treatment can vary from the guidance if the reason is discussed with the patient and recorded in their clinical notes.

We have listed below the organisations in the UK whose methods, opinions and judgements are widely respected as useful and we commend their guidance.

The General Dental Council (**GDC**) is the regulatory body for dentists. A patient can sue a dentist, an employer may sack them but the General Dental Council can stop them working completely so its guidance is the most important. It should be read and digested as a priority by everyone intending to qualify as a dentist in the UK.

https://www.gdc-uk.org/professionals/standards

The Resuscitation Council (**Resus**) is a UK body of medical professionals which sets the standards required for the management of cardio-pulmonary resuscitation in the UK. https://www.resus.org.uk/

The British Dental Association (**BDA**) represents the interests of dentists; it provides advice on clinical, legal and managerial aspects of dentistry. It also organises continual professional development and training and provides meetings, social activities and library facilities.

https://bda.org/

Guidance of Relevance to Oral Surgery at the level of dental qualification examination:

- Preparing for practice Dental team learning outcomes for registration (2015 revised edition) Subsection: Outcomes for dentists. *GDC*

- Standards for Dental Professionals and supplementary guidance documents. *GDC*

- Medical Emergencies *GDC*

- Quality standards for cardiopulmonary resuscitation and training. Primary dental care - Quality standards and Primary dental care - equipment list. *Resus*

- BDA advice Medical Emergencies *BDA*

- BDA advice Infection Control *BDA*

- Management of Acute Dental Problems *SDCEP*

- Guidance on the Extraction of Wisdom Teeth *NICE*

- Management of Dental Patients Taking Anticoagulants or Antiplatelet Drugs *SDCEP*

- Standards for Conscious Sedation in the Provision of Dental Care. The dental faculties of the Royal Colleges of Surgeons and the Royal College of Anaesthetists Report of the Intercollegiate Advisory Committee for Sedation in Dentist *RCS*

- BDA advice Radiation Protection *BDA*

- Antimicrobial Prescribing in Dentistry *CGD*

- Clinical Examination and Record-Keeping *CGD*

- Selection Criteria for Dental Radiography *CGD*

The Scottish Dental Clinical Effectiveness Programme (*SDCEP*) is part of NHS Scotland and provides advice and guidance on good practice in dentistry care liaising with other bodies and taking account of international best practice policies and guidance. http://www.sdcep.org.uk

The National Institute for Health and Care Excellence (*NICE*) is a public body, part of the UK Department of Health which provides advice on health care technologies and clinical care as well as health promotion and social care. https://www.nice.org.uk/

The Royal College of Surgeons of England (*RCS*) provided the first formal qualification in dentistry in the nineteenth century. Its Faculty of Dental Surgery provides some clinical advice, post graduate meetings and post graduate examinations.

https://www.rcseng.ac.uk

The new College of General Dentistry (**CGD**) has taken over the role of the former Faculty of General Dental Practice of the Royal College of Surgeons of England. The faculty published guidelines related to dentistry and these are now available at the College of General Dentistry web site.

https://cgdent.uk/

Guidance of Relevance to Oral Surgery at the level of dental qualification examination (continued):

▪ BDA advice Prescribing and medicines management ***BDA***

• Management of the Palatally Ectopic Maxillary Canine *RCS*

• The Oral Management of Oncology Patients Requiring Radiotherapy, Chemotherapy and/or Bone Marrow Transplantation *RCS*

(All these are available free online)

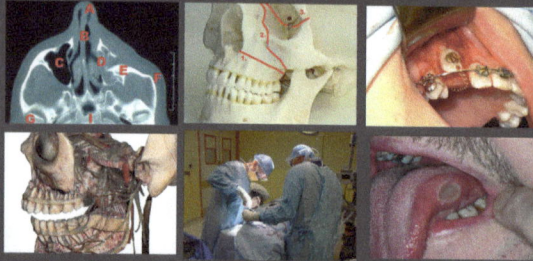

Dentist on the Ward

12th Edition

An Introduction to Oral and Maxillofacial Surgery and Medicine
For Core Trainees in Dentistry

Andrew Sadler and Leo Cheng

Dentist on the Ward provides a concise introduction to oral and maxillofacial surgery for those starting hospital work or previously unfamiliar with the speciality or hospital environment. It will also help in the preparation for undergraduate and non-specialist post-graduate dental examinations.

41 concise chapters provide an introduction to the hospital departments that contribute to the care of oral and maxillofacial patients and guidance on procedures the new appointee may have to carry out.

There are background explanations about the clinical conditions managed by oral and maxillofacial surgeons and their management. This includes oral medicine, and the essential medical information which relates to dental, oral and maxillofacial practice.